How to Manage Chronic Fatigue

Christine Craggs-Hinton, mother of three, followed a career in the civil service until, in 1991, she developed fibromyalgia, a chronic pain condition. Christine took up writing for therapeutic reasons, and has in the past few years produced more than a dozen books for Sheldon Press, including *Living with Fibromyalgia*, *The Chronic Fatigue Healing Diet* and *Coping Successfully with Psoriasis*. Since moving to the Canary Islands, where she has been the resident agony aunt for a local newspaper, she has also taken up fiction writing.

Overcoming Common Problems Series

Selected titles

A full list of titles is available from Sheldon Press,
36 Causton Street, London SW1P 4ST and on our website at
www.sheldonpress.co.uk

The Assertiveness Handbook
Mary Hartley

Assertiveness: Step by step
Dr Windy Dryden and Daniel Constantinou

Backache: What you need to know
Dr David Delvin

Body Language: What you need to know
David Cohen

The Cancer Survivor's Handbook
Dr Terry Priestman

The Candida Diet Book
Karen Brody

The Chronic Fatigue Healing Diet
Christine Craggs-Hinton

The Chronic Pain Diet Book
Neville Shone

Cider Vinegar
Margaret Hills

The Complete Carer's Guide
Bridget McCall

The Confidence Book
Gordon Lamont

Confidence Works
Gladeana McMahon

Coping Successfully with Pain
Neville Shone

Coping Successfully with Panic Attacks
Shirley Trickett

Coping Successfully with Period Problems
Mary-Claire Mason

Coping Successfully with Psoriasis
Christine Craggs-Hinton

Coping Successfully with Ulcerative Colitis
Peter Cartwright

Coping Successfully with Varicose Veins
Christine Craggs-Hinton

Coping Successfully with Your Hiatus Hernia
Dr Tom Smith

Coping Successfully with Your Irritable Bowel
Rosemary Nicol

Coping When Your Child Has Cerebral Palsy
Jill Eckersley

Coping with Age-related Memory Loss
Dr Tom Smith

Coping with Birth Trauma and Postnatal Depression
Lucy Jolin

Coping with Bowel Cancer
Dr Tom Smith

Coping with Candida
Shirley Trickett

Coping with Chemotherapy
Dr Terry Priestman

Coping with Chronic Fatigue
Trudie Chalder

Coping with Coeliac Disease
Karen Brody

Coping with Compulsive Eating
Ruth Searle

Coping with Diabetes in Childhood and Adolescence
Dr Philippa Kaye

Coping with Diverticulitis
Peter Cartwright

Coping with Down's Syndrome
Fiona Marshall

Coping with Dyspraxia
Jill Eckersley

Coping with Eating Disorders and Body Image
Christine Craggs-Hinton

Coping with Epilepsy in Children and Young People
Susan Elliot-Wright

Coping with Family Stress
Dr Peter Cheevers

Coping with Gout
Christine Craggs-Hinton

Coping with Hay Fever
Christine Craggs-Hinton

Coping with Headaches and Migraine
Alison Frith

Overcoming Common Problems Series

Coping with Hearing Loss
Christine Craggs-Hinton

Coping with Heartburn and Reflux
Dr Tom Smith

Coping with Kidney Disease
Dr Tom Smith

Coping with Life after Stroke
Dr Mareeni Raymond

Coping with Macular Degeneration
Dr Patricia Gilbert

Coping with a Mid-life Crisis
Derek Milne

Coping with PMS
Dr Farah Ahmed and Dr Emma Cordle

Coping with Polycystic Ovary Syndrome
Christine Craggs-Hinton

Coping with Postnatal Depression
Sandra L. Wheatley

Coping with Radiotherapy
Dr Terry Priestman

Coping with a Stressed Nervous System
Dr Kenneth Hambly and Alice Muir

Coping with Suicide
Maggie Helen

Coping with Tinnitus
Christine Craggs-Hinton

Coping with Type 2 Diabetes
Susan Elliot-Wright

Coping with Your Partner's Death: Your bereavement guide
Geoff Billings

The Depression Diet Book
Theresa Cheung

Depression: Healing emotional distress
Linda Hurcombe

Depressive Illness
Dr Tim Cantopher

Eating for a Healthy Heart
Robert Povey, Jacqui Morrell and Rachel Povey

Every Woman's Guide to Digestive Health
Jill Eckersley

The Fertility Handbook
Dr Philippa Kaye

The Fibromyalgia Healing Diet
Christine Craggs-Hinton

Free Your Life from Fear
Jenny Hare

Free Yourself from Depression
Colin and Margaret Sutherland

A Guide to Anger Management
Mary Hartley

Heal the Hurt: How to forgive and move on
Dr Ann Macaskill

Helping Children Cope with Anxiety
Jill Eckersley

Helping Children Cope with Grief
Rosemary Wells

How to Approach Death
Julia Tugendhat

How to be a Healthy Weight
Philippa Pigache

How to Beat Pain
Christine Craggs-Hinton

How to Cope with Difficult People
Alan Houel and Christian Godefroy

How to Fight Chronic Fatigue
Christine Craggs-Hinton

How to Get the Best from Your Doctor
Dr Tom Smith

How to Stop Worrying
Dr Frank Tallis

How to Talk to Your Child
Penny Oates

Hysterectomy: Is it right for you?
Janet Wright

The IBS Healing Plan
Theresa Cheung

Letting Go of Anxiety and Depression
Dr Windy Dryden

Living with Angina
Dr Tom Smith

Living with Asperger Syndrome
Dr Joan Gomez

Living with Autism
Fiona Marshall

Living with Bipolar Disorder
Dr Neel Burton

Living with Birthmarks and Blemishes
Gordon Lamont

Living with Crohn's Disease
Dr Joan Gomez

Living with Eczema
Jill Eckersley

Living with Fibromyalgia
Christine Craggs-Hinton

Living with Food Intolerance
Alex Gazzola

Overcoming Common Problems Series

Living with Gluten Intolerance
Jane Feinmann

Living with Grief
Dr Tony Lake

Living with Loss and Grief
Julia Tugendhat

Living with Osteoarthritis
Dr Patricia Gilbert

Living with Osteoporosis
Dr Joan Gomez

Living with Physical Disability and Amputation
Dr Keren Fisher

Living with Rheumatoid Arthritis
Philippa Pigache

Living with Schizophrenia
Dr Neel Burton and Dr Phil Davison

Living with a Seriously Ill Child
Dr Jan Aldridge

Living with Sjögren's Syndrome
Sue Dyson

Living with Type 1 Diabetes
Dr Tom Smith

Losing a Child
Linda Hurcombe

The Multiple Sclerosis Diet Book
Tessa Buckley

Osteoporosis: Prevent and treat
Dr Tom Smith

Overcome Your Fear of Flying
Professor Robert Bor, Dr Carina Eriksen and Margaret Oakes

Overcoming Agoraphobia
Melissa Murphy

Overcoming Anorexia
Professor J. Hubert Lacey, Christine Craggs-Hinton and Kate Robinson

Overcoming Anxiety
Dr Windy Dryden

Overcoming Back Pain
Dr Tom Smith

Overcoming Depression
Dr Windy Dryden and Sarah Opie

Overcoming Emotional Abuse
Susan Elliot-Wright

Overcoming Hurt
Dr Windy Dryden

Overcoming Insomnia
Susan Elliot-Wright

Overcoming Jealousy
Dr Windy Dryden

Overcoming Panic and Related Anxiety Disorders
Margaret Hawkins

Overcoming Procrastination
Dr Windy Dryden

Overcoming Shyness and Social Anxiety
Ruth Searle

Overcoming Tiredness and Exhaustion
Fiona Marshall

Reducing Your Risk of Cancer
Dr Terry Priestman

Safe Dieting for Teens
Linda Ojeda

Self-discipline: How to get it and how to keep it
Dr Windy Dryden

The Self-Esteem Journal
Alison Waines

Simplify Your Life
Naomi Saunders

Sinusitis: Steps to healing
Dr Paul Carson

Stammering: Advice for all ages
Renée Byrne and Louise Wright

Stress-related Illness
Dr Tim Cantopher

Ten Steps to Positive Living
Dr Windy Dryden

Think Your Way to Happiness
Dr Windy Dryden and Jack Gordon

The Thinking Person's Guide to Happiness
Ruth Searle

Tranquillizers and Antidepressants: When to take them, how to stop
Professor Malcolm Lader

The Traveller's Good Health Guide
Dr Ted Lankester

Treating Arthritis Diet Book
Margaret Hills

Treating Arthritis: The drug-free way
Margaret Hills and Christine Horner

Treating Arthritis: More ways to a drug-free life
Margaret Hills

Understanding Obsessions and Compulsions
Dr Frank Tallis

When Someone You Love Has Dementia
Susan Elliot-Wright

When Someone You Love Has Depression
Barbara Baker

Overcoming Common Problems

How to Manage Chronic Fatigue

CHRISTINE CRAGGS-HINTON

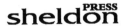
sheldon PRESS

First published in Great Britain in 2010

Sheldon Press
36 Causton Street
London SW1P 4ST

British Library Cataloguing-in-Publication Data
A catalogue record for this book is available from the British Library

ISBN 978-1-84709-064-5

1 3 5 7 9 10 8 6 4 2

Typeset by Fakenham Photosetting Ltd, Fakenham, Norfolk NR21 8NN
Printed in Great Britain by Ashford Colour Press

Produced on paper from sustainable forests

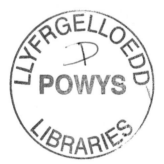

Contents

Introduction   ix

1 Managing your energy   1
2 Putting pacing into practice   15
3 Rest and sleep   28
4 Emotional support   43
5 Diet and nutrition   62
6 Exercise   82
7 Complementary therapies   95

Further reading   105
Useful addresses   106
Index   108

Introduction

Chronic fatigue syndrome (CFS, for short) is a complex condition affecting people of both sexes, though it is more prevalent in women than men. It is defined as chronic (persistent) fatigue which may be severe, sometimes to the point of extreme exhaustion, and which doesn't generally improve after rest. The fatigue can fluctuate throughout the day depending upon physical, physiological and emotional factors. It can also be different from day to day.

Several other symptoms combine with chronic fatigue to make the condition a 'syndrome'. These symptoms may include the following:

- flu-like aching in the muscles and joints, but no swelling;
- other low-grade flu-like symptoms such as sweating and shivering;
- difficulty getting to sleep or waking up very early;
- cognitive problems (also called 'brain fog') – i.e. forgetfulness, memory loss, confusion and difficulty concentrating;
- headaches;
- tender lymph nodes (glands) in the neck and/or armpits;
- dizziness and loss of balance;
- mood swings;
- slurred speech and difficulty finding the right words;
- palpitations;
- feeling sick;
- sensitivity to bright light and loud noise;
- food and chemical sensitivities;
- chronic yeast infections.

As many of the above symptoms can be caused by problems other than CFS, it is important that you seek advice from your GP rather than self-diagnosing.

In 2002, a report by the Department of Health stated that CFS should be recognized as a real, long-lasting illness requiring prompt, accurate and authoritative diagnosis and care by a multidisciplinary team. It added that care should include graded exercise and activity routines, cognitive behavioural therapy and pacing advice. These things are described in this book.

In many cases, the recognition of CFS by the Department of Health as a genuine medical condition signalled the end of disparaging comments (for a few years it was laughingly referred to as 'yuppy flu') and brought with it the first real appreciation of what it must be like to have persistent fatigue, to wake up very tired and to feel so exhausted throughout the day that you are unable to carry out your normal activities. However, there are still plenty of people who can't imagine what it's like to have little or no energy and to be plagued by a myriad of other symptoms – which provides yet another challenge for the person affected. It's a fact that even some GPs fail to accept that CFS is a genuine medical condition, and this is largely because no laboratory tests can, as yet, demonstrate its presence. We can only hope that the condition will soon be verifiable in tests.

So what does it feel like to have CFS? Well, the persistent fatigue is often described as 'like having flu that won't go away'. People with CFS have branded the fatigue as 'overwhelming' and 'like no other type of fatigue'. Rest rarely eases the fatigue and it is nothing like the everyday tiredness that comes after a day's work or a couple of hours of gardening.

CFS has been categorized in the following ways:

- *Mild* – You can perform light tasks and care for yourself. You may be able to work full-time, but need to take some days off sick and can only remain in your job by resting at evenings and weekends.
- *Moderate* – Owing to your levels of fatigue you have probably swapped full-time for part-time work, or have given up employment altogether. You may need an afternoon nap and are more limited in your daily tasks, including caring for yourself.
- *Severe* – Caring for yourself is difficult and you are likely to have memory and concentration problems. You rarely get out of the house, and may need a wheelchair when you do. Any effort causes severe and prolonged exhaustion.
- *Very severe* – For most of the time you are in bed, unable to walk or care for yourself. Your sensitivity to light and noise is pronounced, as are your memory and concentration problems.

The symptoms of CFS have a definite onset – that is, they start at a particular point in time and force you to reduce your activity levels compared with what you were used to. Some people develop the condition after an infection such as glandular fever or the flu virus, but the fatigue is more pronounced than the simple tiredness that often follows the flu. Indeed, persistent enterovirus infections are believed to exist in six out of ten people with CFS – these infections occur in the gastrointestinal tract and sometimes spread to the central nervous system or other parts of the body. Many more viruses are currently under investigation as possible triggers.

As there is no definitive test for CFS, a doctor will normally ask questions about your symptoms before even thinking of making a diagnosis. Many of the symptoms associated with CFS can be indicators of other conditions such as anaemia, liver and kidney problems or an under-active thyroid gland, and therefore blood tests may be ordered. If your doctor diagnoses CFS, you may be offered painkillers such as ibuprofen or paracetamol to ease muscle and joint pain. If depression is one of your symptoms, antidepressants may also be prescribed. Taking such tablets can certainly help you to cope on a day-to-day basis, but they cannot cure the condition. Indeed, until a cure is found you may decide that other more natural treatment options can help you to get more from your life than you otherwise would. Such treatment options are described in detail in this book.

CFS is often described as a sister condition of a chronic pain disorder known as fibromyalgia, from which I have suffered for 18 years. The two conditions have many symptoms in common, including persistent fatigue. I have used the techniques described in this book for many years to cope with my pain and fatigue, and although I am still liable to severe flare-ups if I don't stick to my self-imposed rules, in general I am a million times better than I would have been if I had carried on pushing myself beyond my limits, eating junk food, not exercising, and so on.

If you have a problem with maintaining concentration, it is best to follow the advice given below:

- Don't start reading when you are exhausted already; wait until you feel you can cope with it.
- Only read what you can comfortably manage in one session – two pages, one page, half a page or one paragraph. Using this simple technique should stave off fatigue and help you to absorb what you are reading.
- If possible, alternate reading with a physical activity you find manageable such as doing the washing up or going for a short walk.

Please note that although many doctors refer to the condition as chronic fatigue syndrome (CFS), patients often dislike this term as 'fatigue' is an everyday word which doesn't reflect the severity of the problem. In the UK, patients tend to prefer the term 'myalgic encephalomyelitis' (ME, for short) – 'myalgic' meaning muscle aches and pains and 'encephalomyelitis' meaning inflammation of the brain and spinal cord. However, as research has shown no evidence of such inflammation, doctors are reluctant to use this term.

Because both terms are still in general use, I will refer to the condition as CFS/ME from now on in this book.

Author's note to the reader

This book is intended as a guide to help you cope better emotionally, increase your energy levels and lead a more fulfilling life. It is not a medical book and it is not intended to replace advice from your doctor. If you think you have chronic fatigue syndrome/myalgic encephalomyelitis (CFS/ME) and have not consulted your doctor, please do so.

1

Managing your energy

When you have chronic fatigue syndrome/myalgic encephalomyelitis (CFS/ME), your symptoms can fluctuate so much it is like spending your life on a rollercoaster. Indeed, you are likely to career between periods of intense fatigue (and other symptoms) and relatively smoother times. The smoother times tend not to last very long, however, as it is only too tempting to push yourself too far, with the result that you come to a full stop and need a great deal of rest. Taking a lot of rest when the symptoms subside isn't the answer, either – it unnecessarily reduces muscle tone and joint mobility, and increases negative emotions. Moreover, a cycle of over-activity followed by too much rest is anxiety-provoking and thoroughly demoralizing, making you feel out of control. The best way out of this cycle is to use the technique known as 'pacing', as discussed in this chapter and the next.

Pacing is an energy and lifestyle management strategy through which people with CFS/ME can stabilize their symptoms. By using this strategy, the usual rhythm of over-activity followed by setbacks is often avoided, enabling symptoms to become more stable. It involves not overdoing any type of activity or rest for too long. In time, you learn to balance activity with appropriate rest periods and to live within the limitations imposed by the illness. Activity and appropriate rest periods should be alternated, with the aim of very gradually increasing your activity levels and reducing your rest periods.

It is important that any activity – whether it requires physical, social, mental or emotional effort – is broken up into manageable portions and that, if possible, you switch from one type of activity to another before taking a planned rest. Of course, changing from one activity to another is not always possible, especially if you need to do something time-consuming such as going to the shops. However, if you can do it at least some of the time it can stop you from tiring too quickly.

Note that pacing does not require that you set goals and strive hard to achieve targets. Doing this can be counter-productive, for it is likely to make you push yourself beyond your limits, which of course can result in a sharp rise in fatigue and a need for a long period of rest. Pacing should always be gentle. When you have used the technique very carefully for a length of time, you should find that your body is naturally capable, little by little, of extending your active times.

Another happy side-effect of pacing is the reduction in levels of stress. This means that the rollercoaster car has left the extreme ups and downs of its normal track and has begun gliding smoothly along a lovely flat road. It can be said, then, that symptom stability greatly encourages emotional stability.

As very little research has been carried out to show that pacing is effective as an energy management technique, there is a small amount of controversy about it. However, virtually everyone who uses it properly would gladly tell you how effective it is. Some say that pacing is simply common sense and that it is just a matter of 'listening to your body'. It's a fact, though, that a small proportion of people with CFS/ME have either lost confidence in this ability or experience delayed sensations of fatigue, both of which make pacing difficult to carry out. Delayed sensations of fatigue are discussed below.

Planning your everyday life

Pacing requires that you plan every day of your life for as long as a lack of energy is a problem. Living in this way may seem artificial but it gives back the sense that you are once more in control, which is enormously lifting.

Most people with CFS/ME are inclined to treat the condition the way they would treat any other illness, by resting when they feel bad – which is invariably after doing more than they can cope with. Changing to living a planned life rather than pushing ahead and then reacting to symptoms is often a real challenge, but well worth it when slowly the condition stabilizes and you find yourself with increasing amounts of energy. Moreover, it allows you to understand the cycle of 'flare-ups' followed by the need for rest. A lot of people with CFS/ME view their fluctuations as random – a peculiarity of their illness – but living life according to a schedule can help them to see that these fluctuations virtually always occur after overdoing something, in either a physical or an emotional sense.

Delayed sensations of fatigue

A growing sensation of fatigue warns healthy people that they need to slow down, but this sensation is delayed in a number of people with CFS/ME; the medical term for this is 'faulty perception'. For instance, you may experience no rise in fatigue when you are out doing the shopping, but three to four hours later feel thoroughly drained.

A lack of trustworthy signals at the right time is another good reason for living a planned life. It's certainly a better option than living in response to symptoms, which gets you nowhere at all. Indeed, for people with delayed sensations of fatigue, using the pacing technique is their best chance of making a significant improvement.

Listen to your body

Fortunately, most individuals with CFS/ME still experience normal sensations of increasing fatigue: their problem is that they are not used to tuning into them. The usual reason for this is a lack of trust in what their bodies are trying to tell them – and, unfortunately, it is only too easy to lose trust in your body's signals when you feel worn out anyway for much of the time.

If you still have the ability to listen to your body – whether or not you are used to doing so – and you resolve to be watchful for a rise in symptoms, you will definitely notice them. And so, at the very first signs of increasing fatigue, you should stop what you are doing and take a relaxing break. It's no good being aware that you are growing more tired and having difficulty concentrating when you don't immediately do something about it. Indeed, if you don't act, you will only find yourself feeling terrible, hurting all over and needing a lot more rest than you had bargained for. Moreover, in this situation it is easy to feel disappointed with yourself for allowing yourself to overdo it. Pushing yourself despite growing fatigue also ensures that you delay stabilizing your symptoms and that you put off being able to gradually increase the activities in your daily routine – which is not what you want at all!

For the sake of stability and future improvement, it's vital that you listen to the signals given out by your body. CFS/ME symptoms can escalate very quickly, so you actually need to rest at the very first indications that your body is struggling. If you can take heed of your body's signals throughout the day, you stand a good chance of stabilizing quickly and being able to get far more out of your life in the weeks and months to come.

It is an enormous help if you can spend a few days assessing your limits, writing down each activity you have embarked upon and the category it fell into – whether 'moderate', 'tiring' or 'very tiring' – before you felt the first indications of increasing fatigue. There is information on how to do this in the next few pages.

Identifying your limits

It's hard to live within limits; it's even harder to know where your limits lie. However, having a good idea of your limits is important to the success of the pacing technique.

In order to identify your limits, try very hard to do the following:

- Accept that you feel better or worse depending on your levels of activity.
- Commit to staying within the limits of a planned pacing regime.
- Find the patience to wait – maybe for several months – for your pacing strategy to start increasing your energy levels.
- Muster the self-control required to live a planned life. The effort pays dividends in the end, so is well worth it.

Your base-line

Before you start to list your activities, try to work out where your 'base-line' lies. Your base-line is the minimum you can do in a week, without overdoing rest periods, and it should be mostly comprised of essential activities. If you know that certain essential activities take too much out of you, delegate them to others if at all possible. For example, encourage your children to earn their pocket money by helping you out, and explain to your partner or a parent that if they could kindly take on the heavier work, they'll be rewarded by seeing you a lot less incapacitated.

You may be surprised to learn that for many people their base-line is as low as 25 per cent of what they are used to trying to do – and yes, they feel so ill because they are constantly pushing themselves. If you are wondering how you can possibly do so much less than normal, remember that sticking to the limitations imposed by the illness has the effect of gradually stabilizing your symptoms. This, in turn, allows you slowly but surely to increase the time you are able to spend on different activities and to incorporate further activities into your daily routine. Just as importantly, it allows you to feel better and to be far more positive about your life.

Make an activity list

You are likely to know from experience how you generally respond to certain activities. Therefore, you are likely to have a good idea of how much you can manage to do in one day without provoking an exacerbation of symptoms – and yes, it is probably a lot less than you would ideally like to do. When you feel up to it and with your base-line in mind, use the first page of a notebook to make a list of the things you feel you may be able to manage in a week, as shown in Example 1 on page 6.

As you make your list, keep in mind that you should never carry out an activity you know will create so much fatigue that you'll be exhausted for at least a day afterwards. This will send your pacing plan awry – and the more you fail to stick to it, the more difficult it will be to have another try. If you really have no choice but to carry out a very tiring activity – a hospital appointment, for example – the best way of coping is to ensure that you rest for a few days beforehand and have a very quiet day – or few days – afterwards. (See Chapter 2 for more information on how to cope with taxing events.)

Exercise 1

Included in your list of activities should be a few minutes of very gentle exercise every day. This is vitally important to improving muscle tone, joint mobility and general stamina, all of which are often greatly impacted upon in CFS/ME. Please don't panic at the mention of the word 'exercise'. Chapter 6 guides you through choosing a routine with which you can comfortably cope and shows you how to gradually improve your repertoire.

As I cannot emphasize enough the importance of following an exercise regime, you may find it useful to read Chapter 6 now so that, before you make your activity list, you will have an idea of the exercises you think you can quite easily do. If you are so severely affected by CFS/ME that you spend virtually all your time in bed and feel too awful even to comb your own hair, you may think that exercising is the last thing you should be trying and the last thing you will be capable of doing. This is not the case, however. In the early days of my fibromyalgia I was so incapacitated that I spent all my time in bed and could not even feed myself or look after myself in any way. My means of very slowly working myself out of this state was to perform one or two simple stretching exercises three to four times a day. I remember being unable to put my hands on top of my head when I first tried to stretch my arms, but attempting to very gently reach upwards at regular intervals gradually improved the mobility of my shoulder joints. After about a year, I was able to stretch my arms straight up, high into the air. During that year, I gradually added further stretching exercises to my repertoire and they made a lot of difference to my overall state. I can't say that I didn't overdo it at times – I did, and it invariably set me back. However, I tried to view the setbacks as 'learning experiences', which stopped me from feeling too angry and disappointed with myself.

If your symptoms warn against you performing your exercise routine on a particular day, make sure that you take it up again as soon as your body allows. Always listen to your body. If you feel you have a limited amount of energy one day and it's a choice between exercising and doing the ironing, you really need to choose to exercise. I know it's far from easy to ask other people to do things for you, but if you explain that you are now following a special pacing regime that stands a good chance of making you feel more energized and better in general, they should understand. Alternatively, why not put up with a bit of dust and clutter for a few months, or for however long it takes you to make improvements?

If you can stick to the pacing routine to the best of your ability, you may have occasional setbacks, but in the long term improvement will almost certainly come.

Amanda

Amanda is a 25-year-old young woman who is moderately affected by CFS/ME. Trying to keep in mind her reactions to each hobby or task she had carried out of late, she listed the activities she judged made up her base-line, inclusive of an exercise routine. She then placed an asterisk by the description that best described her response to each.

For a discussion of the activity list of a person with severe symptoms, see pages 10–11.

Example 1: Amanda's activity list

Activity	Manageable	Tiring	Very tiring
Self-care	*		
Making meals	*		
Dusting		*	
Laundry		*	
Ironing			*
Driving		*	
Light shopping			*
Short walk		*	
Reading	*		
Writing short emails	*		
Painting landscapes			*
Gentle exercise routine	*		

Planning the week

When Amanda had finished her activity list, identifying those activities she could manage and those she found tiring or very tiring, she began to rearrange them so that she was only carrying out at the most one very tiring activity a day. For instance, in her activity list, three very tiring activities were identified, one of which she assigned for Mondays, another for Wednesdays and another for Fridays. Of the four tiring activities, she assigned one for Sundays, another for Tuesdays, another for Thursdays and another for Saturdays. In this way they were as separate as she could possibly make them.

Amanda chose a manageable exercise routine with the aim of gradually increasing her repertoire and number of repetitions. If her symptoms were worse than normal on a particular day, she resolved to drop one of her tiring or very tiring activities instead of the exercise routine.

As a result, her 'pacing chart' looked something like Example 2.

Example 2: Amanda's pacing chart

Day	Activities
Mondays	Self-care, exercise routine, making meals, reading, light shopping
Tuesdays	Self-care, exercise routine, making meals, reading, writing emails, laundry
Wednesdays	Self-care, exercise routine, making meals, reading, ironing
Thursdays	Self-care, exercise routine, making meals, reading, writing emails, short walk
Fridays	Self-care, exercise routine, making meals, reading, painting landscapes
Saturdays	Self-care, exercise routine, making meals, reading, writing emails, driving
Sundays	Self-care, exercise routine, making meals, reading, dusting

Rest periods in between

When devising your own pacing chart, it's important that you remember the need to rest between tiring and very tiring activities. Obviously, the most tiring of activities require longer rest periods afterwards than the less tiring. Every time you fail to rest sufficiently after a tiring or very tiring activity you build up your levels of fatigue, which will eventually bring you to a full stop. Prolonged rest is then the only way out, and so you are back on that rollercoaster.

It is best, then, to rest only for as long as you think you need to, and no longer at all – unless you are stock-piling energy to cope with a taxing event.

Alternate tiring and less tiring activities

During your day, it's important to alternate tiring or very tiring activities with more manageable ones. Saving your most demanding of activities until late in the day means you are working on a depleted energy tank, which will wear you out a lot faster than it might have done earlier in the day. In other words, it is advisable to get on with your most taxing activities when you are feeling your best. As following a daily exercise routine is of paramount importance, it is advisable to carry this out early in the day.

When there are several tiring or very tiring activities

If, when you come to compile your own activity list, it flags up lots of tiring and very tiring activities, the rearrangement (pacing chart) will probably still show that you expect to carry out two or more of such activities on more than one day – maybe even every day of the week. In this case, it is strongly recommended that you think hard about what it is actually *essential* that you do – in other words, that you find your base-line, as discussed on page 4. The whole idea of pacing is that you not only spread out the more difficult of your activities but also drop certain activities – with the exception of an exercise regime – until your symptoms lessen and you feel more energized.

If you think it's not possible for you to drop even the most demanding of your activities – say, because you live alone – remember that there are solutions to almost everything in life. You might not like asking family and friends to help out, but for the sake of your health and the chance of improvement, it needs to be done. If you can afford a cleaner, I would strongly advise that you employ one. A friend or relative who helps out may even be entitled to claim benefit from Social Services, or you may be able to claim. Any benefit you receive is intended as a purse from which you can pay for cleaners, gardeners, taxi fares and any other help you need. For people who have no one at all to help out, it's vital that you speak to your doctor about help from Social Services and Occupational Therapy departments.

If you live with a partner and children aged eight and over, you really need to ask them for help with the activities you find most taxing. For instance, you could ask your partner to help with house-work and to either do the shopping or accompany you to the shops so that he or she can do most of the carrying, and maybe even the driving. Also, there's nothing wrong with asking children of eight and over to dry the dishes, and do a little dusting or hoovering. Children of 13 and older (or even younger, depending on the individual child's maturity) could be taught how to do the washing and ironing and how to make certain meals – in this way, you are not only helping yourself, you are also preparing your children for adult life. Of course, children are always more willing to help if you remember to thank them and praise what they do, and ensure that they still have enough time to themselves. Children under eight years old should not be expected to do too much housework, but can run upstairs to bring you a jumper, help to whisk the Yorkshire pudding batter, bring you a drink of water and so on – simple jobs that make them feel useful and that are a help to you.

When enjoyable activities are very tiring

So what about the activities you really enjoy, but which make you feel exhausted and exacerbate your other symptoms? In Example 1, I have given painting landscapes as my illustration, but it could be card-making, writing poetry, tapestry-work, model-making, playing the piano or tinkering with the car – anything that provides enjoyment and a sense of satisfaction.

Using my example of painting landscapes, there are a variety of art materials to choose from, the most popular being watercolour paints and oils. Most watercolour artists use the 'wet on wet' technique, which requires that they complete the painting in one session. Obviously, if you become aware of increasing fatigue while you are only part way through such a 'one-shot' hobby, remember that your pacing plan could be sent seriously awry if you push on regardless. Instead, be strong and put your brushes in water straight away, resting then until you feel stronger. You should be able to revive the painting by simply spraying it with water at a later date. If you have managed to complete the painting without immediately exacerbating your symptoms, don't forget to assess your response in the following few hours in case you experience a delayed response. If you do encounter a rise in fatigue – whether it be during or after the activity – your best options are either to swap the activity for one less demanding or to give it up until you have built up more energy.

Going back to the example, if you use oil paints it is best to build your painting over several sessions so there's less risk of you over-doing it – and of course you should monitor your reactions as you go. You will find that you can 'spread the load' in this way with many other forms of craft-work. Doing something pleasurable raises levels of endorphins – the body's natural feel-good chemicals – and so can be a great emotional boost. It's therefore important that you indulge in as many enjoyable activities in your week as you can comfortably manage.

Identify activities which energize you

Many people with CFS/ME unwittingly carry out normal everyday activities which provide a boost and so energize them. The key is to identify these feel-good activities and give them priority. For instance, when Amanda thought about it, she realized that taking a shower made her feel fresh and revitalized, so she made it a point to include a daily shower in her self-care regime. She also realized that chatting to her partner had an energizing effect, as did writing emails to her friends and browsing around city department stores on a Saturday. She therefore made a few changes to her pacing chart.

Example 3: Amanda's improved pacing chart

Day	Activities
Mondays	Self-care (including taking a shower), exercise routine, making meals, reading, writing emails, light shopping
Tuesdays	Self-care (including taking a shower), exercise routine, making meals, reading, writing emails, laundry
Wednesdays	Self-care (including taking a shower), exercise routine, making meals, reading, writing emails, ironing
Thursdays	Self-care (including taking a shower), exercise routine, making meals, reading, writing emails, short walk
Fridays	Self-care (including taking a shower), exercise routine, making meals, reading, writing emails, painting landscapes
Saturdays	Self-care (including taking a shower), exercise routine, making meals, reading, writing emails, driving, looking around department stores
Sundays	Self-care (including taking a shower), exercise routine, making meals, reading, writing emails, dusting

Mark

Mark, 42, is severely affected by CFS/ME, which means that his activity list is quite different from Amanda's. For Mark there are elements of self-care that he is unable to carry out at all. His list, therefore, breaks down self-care into its different components, as shown below. He has also included other activities he thinks he can manage if they are spread out sufficiently, inclusive of his very gentle exercise routine.

Example 4: Mark's activity list

Activity	Manageable	Tiring	Very tiring
Taking a shower			*
Washing hands and face		*	
Brushing teeth	*		
Getting dressed			*
Combing hair		*	
Making a light lunch		*	
Light dusting			*
Reading		*	
Watching TV	*		
Listening to music	*		
Talking to visitors			*
Gentle exercise routine	*		

When Mark had finished spreading out his most tiring activities throughout the week, his pacing chart ended up like this:

Example 5: Mark's pacing chart

Day	Activities
Mondays	Take a shower, brush teeth, comb hair, exercise routine, read, watch TV, listen to music
Tuesdays	Wash hands and face, brush teeth, comb hair, exercise routine, light dusting, read, watch TV, listen to music
Wednesdays	Wash hands and face, brush teeth, comb hair, exercise routine, make a light lunch, read, watch TV, listen to music
Thursdays	Take a shower, brush teeth, comb hair, get dressed, exercise routine, watch TV, listen to music
Fridays	Wash hands and face, brush teeth, comb hair, exercise routine, talk to visitors, watch TV, listen to music
Saturdays	Take a shower, brush teeth, comb hair, exercise routine, make a light lunch, read, watch TV, listen to music
Sundays	Wash hands and face, brush teeth, comb hair, get dressed, exercise routine, talk to visitors, watch TV, listen to music

When Mark thought about it, he was surprised to realize that there was an activity which he, too, found energizing. He is a great fan of hard rock music and feels lifted after listening to bands such as Led Zeppelin, AC/DC, Guns N' Roses, Metallica and Deep Purple. His pacing chart already included listening to music, but he made a point of ensuring that it was hard rock.

Although he finds talking to visitors very tiring, he was able to acknowledge that chatting to his wife gave him a lift, too. The couple therefore made a promise to each other that they would spend at least an hour of quality time together during weekdays, and even longer at weekends. When Mark considered the other people in his life, he recalled that his best friend had a great sense of humour and always made him laugh. As this, too, had an energizing effect, he encouraged his friend to visit more frequently, telling him honestly that he cheered him up.

Mark has always loved cooking, but at the time of preparing his activity list and pacing chart was not able to do more than put together a light meal such as beans on toast, a sandwich or scrambled eggs. Being unable to carry out an enjoyable activity made him feel quite upset, but he cheered up when he realized that by pacing himself he would build up energy and probably be able to start cooking at some point in the future.

Keeping a record of your emotional state

When you have finalized your pacing chart, you should congratulate yourself! This would not be an easy task for a healthy person, never mind someone with limited energy and a myriad of other symptoms. However, as stress uses up energy and compromises your immune system, it's a good idea to make a note of your present emotional state before you start following the chart. At the end of each week, you should then once more describe in words the way you are feeling.

Below are Amanda's notes of her weekly emotional state.

Example 6: Amanda's emotional state

- *Prior to starting the pacing technique* – Just about everything makes me wiped out and tearful. There are so many things I can't do and so I feel useless. I'm sure people think I'm not trying to help myself and I could scream at them sometimes. When I'm in the middle of doing something and know I can't finish it, I feel so frustrated. Why am I like this? Why can't I be normal like everyone else?
- *End of Week 1* – It isn't easy to follow the chart. I can see already, though, that sticking to it will help me. I didn't realize that pushing myself was having such a negative effect and it's nice to be slightly more stable. I did make one or two mistakes, but I'm trying to learn from them. I'm feeling tentatively optimistic.

- *End of Week 2* – Sticking to the regime is quite boring, but I realize how essential it is. I never liked telling my sister that I was exhausted and needed to lie down, but this week I just said it and curled up on the sofa. She actually looked concerned and asked if she could do anything for me – that's a first! I'm starting to feel more empowered.
- *End of Week 3* – Because James has been doing the supermarket shopping, I've actually found that I can paint an entire landscape in one go – it doesn't matter that I'm using smaller sheets of paper than before I got ill. I was incredibly proud of the painting I produced, and while doing it I was able to concentrate better and for once didn't feel the need to rush. What a buzz!

As you can see, Amanda's physical and emotional progress is surprisingly fast – a fact of which she may not have been so aware had she not written down her feelings. She's gradually building up her stamina levels and learning that she can swap and change her activities depending upon how she feels. The notes she makes at the end of each week help her to see that her state of mind is becoming more positive, and that in itself is a boost.

Someone like Mark, who is severely affected, is likely to suffer more setbacks and take more time to see improvements than someone like Amanda. However, as long as he tries hard to stick to his pacing chart and the general rules of pacing he can only gain in confidence and stamina.

Making your own charts

If you wish, you can make your own activity list using the following headings:

Activity   Manageable   Tiring   Very tiring

For your pacing chart, use two columns under the following headings:

Day   Activities

Then record your weekly emotional state. Here's a suggested layout:

Prior to starting the pacing technique:

End of Week 1:

End of Week 2:

End of Week 3:

End of Week 4:

End of Week 5:

End of Week 6:

2

Putting pacing into practice

It is believed that pacing offers the best chance of improvement for someone with CFS/ME, particularly when combined with the other techniques mentioned in this book. So is it really possible to keep to the activities on your pacing chart? And how do you gradually increase your activity levels without causing flare-ups? To help you with these things, several strategies are outlined in this chapter.

Keeping a record of your reactions

Keeping records of your reactions to *all* of your activities, whether you have classed them on your activity list as 'manageable', 'tiring' or 'very tiring', can be greatly beneficial. Indeed, the solid evidence of words on paper will help you to grasp that something you did caused a flare-up of symptoms, and to understand that it wasn't simply a quirk of your illness. Keeping records is also a great motivator, for it encourages you to aim for a life with greatly reduced symptoms. It helps you to stick to a routine, too.

Below are the records of one week in the life of Tara, a 32-year-old woman who is moderately affected by CFS/ME and has stopped working because of her ill-health. After compiling her activity list, Tara worked out her pacing chart to include not more than one very tiring activity per day – and now, using the pacing chart as her guide, she is keen to see the results of her efforts at pacing herself.

Tara begins by keeping a record of her reactions, week by week, in the order shown below:

1 She makes a note of each activity immediately after carrying it out. (She feels well enough to list each of her self-care activities under 'self-care'.)
2 After each activity, she rests for as long as she feels she needs to (see page 3 for more information on getting the right amount of rest between activities).
3 She records her reactions to each activity at the end of each day. (If she thinks she may not be able to remember back that long, she scribbles her reaction in pencil, keeping in mind that the true

reaction may be delayed and she may need to change what she's written.)

Example 7: Tara's records of her reactions, at the end of Week 1

Day	Activity	Reaction
Monday	Self-care	Felt no more tired than normal afterwards
	Exercise routine	ditto
	Changed the bedding	ditto
	Did the laundry	ditto
	Walked to the local shops	ditto
Tuesday	Self-care	Felt no more tired than normal afterwards
	Exercise routine	ditto
	Did the ironing	ditto
	Prepared food for dinner	ditto
	Drove to pay a bill	ditto
Wednesday	Self-care	Felt no more tired than normal afterwards
	Exercise routine	ditto
	Hoovered carpets	ditto
	Went for a short walk	ditto
	Mother visited	ditto
Thursday	Self-care	Felt no more tired than normal afterwards
	Exercise routine	ditto
	Wrote a letter	ditto
	Cleaned the windows	Felt exhausted afterwards and had to spend the remainder of the day in bed
Friday	Self-care	Felt exhausted afterwards so took a long rest
	Exercise routine	Felt exhausted afterwards so spent the remainder of the day in bed
Saturday	Basic self-care only	Felt exhausted afterwards and spent virtually all day in bed
Sunday	Basic self-care only	Felt tired afterwards, but after a longer rest than normal, began to feel better

On looking back over her week, it was clear to Tara that cleaning the windows had been her downfall. Rather than cutting out the activity altogether, she decided to amend her pacing chart. As a result, she planned to clean one window at a time in place of another activity, rather than going through half the house in one go. She asked for help with cleaning the larger glass patio doors.

Do you need to amend your pacing chart?

When you start to record your own reactions you, too, may find that you need to amend your pacing chart. In fact, it may be necessary to amend it several times before you find your base-line of activity, as discussed in Chapter 1. A reminder: if you try to carry out more than the bare minimum of what you can do, it's unlikely that your symptoms will stabilize.

Making your own records of your reactions

Just as Tara did, use a fresh page to note down each activity immediately after finishing it – these are the activities you have already chosen for your pacing chart. Sticking to these activities creates routine, which in turn eliminates the need to make decisions about which activities you may or may not be able to manage. However, if you find you are struggling with your pacing routine after a week or so of attempting to follow it, you need to reassess your daily activities. All being well, you will be able to find your base-line and your symptoms will gradually stabilize. In time, you should be able to add extra activities to your regime – but don't worry about that for now.

You may wish to use the headings below when keeping your own records. As your response to certain activities may have a delayed onset, it is best to write down your reactions at the end of each day, as mentioned earlier. Only leave your report for the next day if you are feeling too tired at the time, and try not to postpone writing down your reactions on a regular basis. Obviously, it is not always easy to clearly remember the details of your activities and reactions after a passage of time.

Week 1

Day   *Activity*   *Reaction*

Week 2

Day   *Activity*   *Reaction*

Week 3

Day   *Activity*   *Reaction*

Week 4

Day   Activity   Reaction

Week 5

Day   Activity   Reaction

Week 6

Day   Activity   Reaction

Discuss how you are doing

You can also help yourself by discussing your progress and setbacks with another person – your partner or a parent, for example – using the records of your reactions for reference. Feeling that you are accountable to someone else helps you to stop pushing yourself beyond your limits.

Read back your records

It's a good idea to review the records of your reactions at the end of each week. In this way it is often surprising to realize just how much progress you have made – progress you may not have appreciated if you had not checked back. The evidence of how well pacing is working for you should then spur you into continuing your schedule.

Have patience

Looking back at your records will also help you to find the patience required to stay within your limits. Rather than seeing months of routine stretching ahead of you, try to focus on one day at a time. If possible, avoid the temptation to hope for a fast improvement. No one can say how long it will take a certain person to start reaping the rewards – we all have different metabolisms and our bodily systems are affected in different ways. Therefore, two people with CFS/ME who appear to be similarly affected may respond to pacing in totally disparate ways.

Avoiding the 'push and crash' cycle

One of the basic rules of pacing is never to over-exert yourself after sensing that you are running low on energy. It is often tempting to continue an activity because it's giving you immediate pleasure and to ignore the niggling worry at the back of your mind that you are overdoing it. For instance, Philip enjoys war games, a hobby which in- volves painting miniature lead soldiers, reproducing their uniforms in painstaking perfection. In his activity chart he has allocated one hour twice a week to this, knowing from experience that spending longer than this on it can lead him into difficulties. However, he gets such a buzz from his hobby that on Week 4 of his pacing regime he overlooks the fact that he's going over his hour. Indeed, he pushes himself to one and a half hours before deciding to leave his figures to dry and take a rest.

Being tempted to overdo things

Unfortunately, people with fatigue and pain problems are constantly tempted to push themselves beyond their limits. There may be several different reasons for this, as shown below:

- You may push yourself because you have visitors coming and want the house to be clean and tidy.
- You are enjoying a particular activity so much that you don't want to stop.
- You believe that this time you'll be lucky and the fatigue won't catch up with you.
- You don't want to overburden other people in your life.
- You make an effort to keep up with others so you don't feel weak and useless.
- There is no one else to carry out certain tasks so you feel you have no choice but to do them yourself.
- Other people in your life don't understand your limitations and expect you to do a certain amount.

Invariably, however, pushing yourself is followed by a crash. For instance, after Philip had spent longer than his allotted time painting his lead figures, he felt so exhausted he was unable even to concentrate on watching TV. Indeed, he could only lie in bed feeling terrible, angrily demanding of himself why he had thought he could get away with it.

Visualize the outcome

Perhaps the most effective way of avoiding the push and crash cycle is to use the technique of visualization. It certainly works for me. Visualization involves mentally picturing the consequences if you go beyond your limits. You know from overdoing things in the past how ill, angry and miserable it makes you, so you should try to visualize this the moment you realize you are in danger of pushing yourself too far.

When Philip had recovered enough that he could get back to his pacing regime and once more began painting his lead soldiers, he was again tempted to carry on for longer than an hour. As soon as he used the visualization technique, however, he could see how bad he would feel if he allowed himself to go on, and therefore he stuck rigidly to his one-hour time limit, knowing that in the weeks and months to come he would have built up enough stamina to spend longer on his hobby.

If, from time to time, you overdo things before your body is ready, you are likely to be more aware than ever that the consequences are the result of straying from the plan.

Self-talk

When you are tempted to ignore your boundaries, there's usually a little voice in your head saying, 'I can get away with it this time – I don't feel too bad,' or 'I feel fine today so I think I've recovered a lot of my stamina.' The best way to see the truth of the situation is to conjure up another little voice saying, 'Improvement is very gradual so I can't be making a sudden recovery,' or 'Pushing myself is just not worth the flare-up I'll no doubt have afterwards. I can finish this another day.'

If you push yourself beyond your limits too often, you risk being thrown back to square one. This applies no matter how much improvement you have made – an improvement which may have taken you months to achieve. It is therefore vital that you are firm in using visualization and positive self-talk to prevent this from happening.

Self-forgiveness

When you do happen to forget all about visualization and positive self-talk, you will probably experience an exacerbation of symptoms, setting back your progress a few days or weeks. Beating yourself up about this is not going to help, however, and you should try hard not to do it. Instead, be forgiving with yourself and content yourself with the knowledge that you'll learn from the experience. If you need a little positive motivation, look back over your records to remind yourself of your progress from the early days. Try to have patience, and you'll soon be back on the road to recovery.

Coping with special occasions

Life is never straightforward for any of us. You may successfully keep to a routine in your day-to-day life, but special occasions such as weddings, birthday parties and Christmas celebrations can threaten your new-found stability. Fortunately, there are strategies which can help you cope, meaning you don't always have to avoid an event you might otherwise have enjoyed. Of course, there may be times when your symptoms are too severe for you to even contemplate attending the event, particularly in the early days of carrying out the pacing technique.

The enjoyment factor

If your condition is not yet stable and you know the event in question would put you in bed for a period afterwards, don't even think about attending – and certainly don't let yourself be pressured into it. On the other hand, if your symptoms are stable or starting to stabilize, it is useful to take the enjoyment factor into account. For instance, try asking yourself if this is the type of event you might have enjoyed if you didn't have CFS/ME, or whether it's an event you would, in the past, have found tedious. If the latter is the case, again don't even think about attending – it just isn't worth it at this stage. However, if the former is the case yet you don't fancy attending the event, try to ascertain whether you are unnecessarily over-protecting yourself when, with extra rest and so on, you could probably cope with the event and get pleasure from being there. It's important that you read Chapter 4 for advice on coping strategies for taxing events.

The fear factor

You may perhaps have reached the stage where the mere thought of doing something outside your normal sphere fills you with dread. Sadly, this mindset is not conducive to improvement as the whole idea of pacing is that, once stability is achieved, you can gradually extend the parameters of your routine (as discussed later in this chapter).

If you regularly find yourself worrying that a flare-up may hold you back and so avoid activities you may otherwise have found pleasurable, you may need additional help from a cognitive behavioural therapist. (Some of the main teachings of cognitive behavioural therapy (CBT) are outlined in Chapter 4.) CBT is excellent for providing you with a more positive mindset and thus enabling you to make the necessary preparations for coping with taxing events. The following section on taking extra rest should help you, too.

Extra rest

Assuming you have chosen to attend a particular event – one you would find enjoyable if you were in good health – it's possible to ward off an exacerbation of symptoms by taking more rest than normal beforehand. This applies after the event, too. It is sensible to prepare for the event a few days in advance, actually doubling the amount of time you would normally rest and thus storing up your energy reserves. When the event is over, commit yourself to resting for as long as it takes until you feel well enough to continue your pacing regime. Hopefully, you will have prepared sufficiently for the event and looked after yourself during it (see below and Chapter 4), as a result of which you may not need to rest for too long afterwards.

If at all possible, look for an opportunity to rest during the event, too. For instance, I recently attended my son's wedding and was able to return to my house to lie down for an hour between the actual ceremony and the start of the speeches. This made all the difference to my pain and fatigue levels, allowing me to enjoy the occasion. It also helped that my son and daughter-in-law thoughtfully held the reception at a venue quite near to my house. They made sure that I didn't miss out on the wedding breakfast either, as they arranged buffet-style food rather than a sit-down meal. I was therefore able to enjoy the food on my return to the venue.

Of course, not all relatives and friends can be expected to plan their special occasion around the needs of one guest. Consequently, I would strongly advise that you get into the habit of looking for ways to make the event in question less risky for you. Explaining your limitations to your hosts is a good starting point.

Explain your limitations

I have always found that I cope better with special occasions if I quietly inform the people around me that I have limits to which I must stick, for the sake of my future improvement. These people are then not surprised or disappointed if I decide to leave early or ask if I can rest on a bed for an hour. They may even schedule an activity requiring physical or mental agility for the period when you are taking a rest.

When to increase your activity levels

Some experts advise that you increase your activity levels very slightly every few days. This is fine if you feel you are coping well with your regime, but not if you are only just coping. Obviously, if you are floundering at all, you need to re-think your activities, delegating the more demanding tasks to other people and perhaps even increasing your rest periods. It is far better to start your pacing regime doing too little than to struggle and risk staying on that rollercoaster.

In reality, no other person can tell you when you are ready to increase your activity levels. No one but you truly knows how you are feeling and how you are responding to your regime as it stands. It is advisable that you wait until you are stable for 10–14 days at the very least before you try raising the stakes.

Selecting activities to recommence or extend

When you think you are ready to recommence an activity you had previously dropped or to extend an activity you are already carrying out, make sure that it's one you would class as 'manageable' – you stand more chance of success in this way. If the activity is also something you enjoy doing, so much the better. Being able to successfully incorporate an old activity into your routine will give you a psychological boost, as will lengthening the time you are already spending on a particular undertaking. On the other hand, being unsuccessful and experiencing a flare-up of symptoms can increase frustration and make you wonder if you will ever improve. For this reason, it is essential that you really do feel confident that you are ready to move forward.

Listen to your body

As increasing activity levels is often a matter of trial and error, it's vital that you listen to the signals your body is sending out – this is also discussed on page 3. For example, after managing to stabilize his symptoms, 24-year-old Connor decided to try extending an activity he found enjoyable though rather demanding: spending more time communicating with friends on Facebook, an internet networking site. Consequently, after spending his usual half-hour on Facebook, he made a point of assessing how he was feeling every couple of minutes. At the very first sign of mounting fatigue or mental tiredness he stopped what he was doing and rested. In this way, he was gradually able to build up his levels of activity. You, too, can do this by being aware of a slight increase in symptoms before they rise to unmanageable levels – don't forget that symptoms often increase very quickly. The rise in symptoms should subside after sufficient rest, but if you need more rest than before you increased your time on the activity, you have either extended your time too much or are not quite ready to implement that increase.

As mentioned on page 3, some people have faulty perception and so experience delayed signals from their bodies. If this is the case with you, it is best to increase your time on particular activities only very gradually. For example, 47-year-old Ruth gets pleasure from seeing her house spick and span, so committed herself to spending 30 minutes a day on housework. After a stable two weeks she tried raising that to 45 minutes, but an exacerbation of symptoms later on in that first day told Ruth that 45 minutes was too long. She waited until her symptoms were once again stable, then increased her housework time by just two or three minutes every other day, and found she coped well with that. Over the next few months she was able to maintain a slow increase in time spent on housework and other activities, provided that she pulled back immediately if she felt she was overdoing it.

Finding easier ways to do things

There are ways of carrying out certain activities that can make life a little easier, as described in this section. Don't forget, however, that before undertaking any activity you must first assess whether or not you are up to it. Try not to take chances, and don't be afraid to delegate. Asking for help does not signify weakness on your part; asking for help takes guts and is an essential part of coping with CFS/ME.

Plan meals in advance

Save time and energy by preparing a few meals in advance and storing them in the freezer to microwave later on. For example, Ruth and her husband enjoy chicken dinners so she is in the habit of roasting two chickens at once and preparing enough vegetables for a total of ten meals. She and her partner are thus able to eat these pre-prepared meals whenever she is feeling over-tired. Connor, who is mentioned on page 23, is single and not yet well enough to cook, so he regularly asks his mother/sister/best friend to kindly prepare several meals for him in advance.

Several types of foods can be frozen until required. For example, Ruth makes a large dish of lasagne in one go and freezes half of it for re-heating at a later date. She also makes a big pan of beef stew and freezes what's left of it for later on.

I wouldn't normally recommend purchasing microwave meals as they tend to contain a lot of fat and artificial additives. However, I see nothing wrong with storing several in your freezer for use in emergencies. Look out for the 'healthy eating' options.

Use energy-saving devices

Investing in energy-saving devices is well worth the initial outlay. For example, long-handled 'reachers' are very useful, as are 'shoppers' (on wheels), hands-free telephones, electric can-openers, jar-openers that grip, electric carving knives, juicers and food processors.

Maintain mobility

Because maintaining one position for an extended period tires the muscles, try to be as mobile as possible when you are carrying out an activity. For example, if you are peeling potatoes at the sink, keep stretching and shifting position.

Sitting for long periods

There may be times when you need to sit for long periods, such as when waiting to see the doctor or dentist, watching a play or film, or attending a family gathering. However, as sitting in one position can create a great deal of fatigue, it is best to do the following:

- If possible, sit in a chair which supports your entire back. (Chairs which look comfortable are not necessarily the most supportive.) Your chosen chair should have adequate lumbar support and arm rests, and it should seat you higher than a standard armchair. The added height makes it easier for you to stand up.
- Ensure you adopt the correct sitting posture. Your bottom should be tucked well into the back of the seat, with your spine supported by the back of the chair. Your head should sit directly on top of your shoulders, so that your body carries its weight. Allowing your head to droop forward puts your neck muscles under a lot of strain and encourages fatigue.
- Place a small cushion in the hollow of your back, around the level of your waist, to encourage good posture. If you are going to a place where there may not be cushions, take a small one with you – I have done this for many years. If it's summer and/or you are going to a place where you know you'll be warm, simply place your jacket or a jumper/cardigan in the hollow of your back.
- Get up and walk around at regular intervals. If you are in someone's home, explain that sitting for too long can tire your muscles, so you need to keep breaking it up. If you are at the theatre or cinema, try to purchase seats at the end of a row. You will not then disturb people as you make regular trips to the loo, the bar, the confectionery kiosk – anywhere so long as you are breaking up the stress on your muscles. If you are waiting to see your doctor or the dentist, again get up and walk around as often as you can. Peruse the notice boards, take a couple of quick trips to the loo or stand looking out of the window for a while ... Don't worry about drawing attention to yourself. Keeping your levels of fatigue under control is of far more importance. If you are at home, remember not to sit for prolonged periods.
- When you need to sit at a desk, use a good chair and bring your work closer to eye level. You can achieve this by using a lap desk or a drafting table. Place frequently used work materials within easy reach, remove the things you don't use and tilt your head back every now and again to compensate for prolonged forward positioning. Also, take regular breaks. If you have a lot of paperwork to get

through, keep getting up and walking around – and remember not to overdo it!

Washing up, preparing vegetables, and so on

Leaning over kitchen work surfaces for prolonged periods can stress the neck and back muscles and so encourage fatigue. It is therefore best to do the following:

- Move as close to the work surface as possible to encourage proper posture.
- Stand tall, making sure to tilt your head and tuck in your chin.
- Place a wooden box on the work surface to bring the work closer (maybe someone keen on DIY could make you one).
- Take regular breaks.

Doing the shopping

When you are shopping, it is best to do the following:

- Park the car as close as possible to the supermarket.
- Carry items close to your body. Most Americans have the right idea where shopping is concerned – they wrap their arms around their packages. Carrying close to the body disperses the strain.
- Limit the amount you carry at one time – making two journeys carrying a lighter load is better than making one journey carrying a heavy load.
- Use a shopping trolley on wheels.
- Take someone with you to share the load.
- Delegate the job to someone else until you are feeling better.

Lifting a bulky object off the floor

When lifting, you should be careful to ensure that the strain is taken by your legs rather than your back. The golden rule is, therefore, LNB – Legs, Not Back. Remember, too, that you must assess, first of all, whether you are really up to lifting. If you choose to go ahead, it is best to keep to the following:

- Plant your feet about 30 cm (12 in) or so apart. A wide base helps maintain correct alignment.
- Keeping your back straight, bend your knees until you are resting on your haunches. Place your arms around the object.
- Push upwards with your legs in order to raise it from the ground.
- If possible, break the load into smaller portions. Where laundry is concerned, it is safer to lift a few items at a time, carrying them close

to your body (perhaps over your arm if the items are dry) to the washing machine/tumble drier/clothes airer.

- If the object is larger than a laundry basket, get someone to help.

3

Rest and sleep

Anyone who doesn't have CFS/ME should first imagine how it might feel to have slept very poorly for several consecutive nights, and then try to imagine feeling like that for the majority of the time. This is what it's like to have CFS/ME, but with the addition of numerous other troublesome symptoms. Impaired sleep is strongly associated with CFS/ME, and finding a way to sleep better can improve matters considerably. Resting properly during daytime relaxation periods can also set you on the road to recovery – however, not everyone knows how to get good rest in today's stress-filled society.

As resting properly and effectively during the day is just as intrinsic to the pacing technique as getting good sleep at night, I will discuss this first.

How to get good daytime rest

When we need to rest during the day, most of us believe that slumping in front of the TV for an hour will suffice. This may be the case for a healthy person whose muscles don't tire easily and who can cope with being stretched or scrunched, but it is certainly not the case if you have CFS/ME, particularly if you are severely affected. However, when you take proper rest during the day, lying down flat on a comfortable and supportive surface, you will soon find that this makes a great difference to how active you can be and how quickly you can improve.

Resting with your eyes open, while lying down, is a great way to physically relax and mentally unwind, as discussed below.

Awareness meditation

Relaxing without closing your eyes is known as 'awareness meditation'. The term relates to the state of being aware of your life and surroundings while at the same time entering a deeply relaxed place. To use this type of meditation, follow these instructions:

1 Go into a warm room where you know you won't be disturbed for as long as you need to rest. Ensure that the room is not too bright.

(You may need to pull the curtains and switch on a small table lamp to create a restful atmosphere.)

2 Lie on your back on a supportive surface, such as a mattress, and make yourself comfortable.

3 Deliberately relax all your muscles, starting at the top with your face and neck and ending with your feet and toes.

4 Don't look around too much. If you wish, try to loosely focus on one particular object without actually thinking about it. You will get better at this with practice.

5 As thoughts pass through your mind, don't hang on to them. Simply allow them to float away. If there is a problem in your life at the moment, don't let yourself pay attention to it. Once again, practice should soon make this skill come as second nature.

6 Stay in the same general position. If you start fidgeting or changing position it's usually because you are mentally focusing on something. If this is so, relax all your muscles once more and allow your conscious mind to drift.

7 If a noise of some kind is disturbing your relaxation, wear earplugs or listen to calming music through headphones. Using tape cassettes, CDs, iPods or MP3 players is better than listening to the radio because of the lack of advertisements or announcements.

8 If your eyelids start to feel droopy, open them, loosely focus again on an object and recommence the whole process. You may occasionally fall asleep during this procedure, which is okay if you are able to sleep at night. However, if you have difficulty sleeping or wake unrefreshed after napping during the day, make a conscious effort not to drop off.

The 'deep breathing' technique

The long-term frustration and anxiety generally linked with CFS/ME commonly leads to chronic stress, the state of being constantly 'on alert'. The physiological changes associated with this state – a fast heart-rate, shallow breathing and muscular tension – often persist over a long period, making relaxation very difficult. As chronic stress can lead to nerviness, hypertension, irritability and depression, it's beneficial to perform a deep breathing exercise at least once a day.

Testing your breathing

In normal breathing, we take oxygen from the atmosphere down into our lungs. The diaphragm contracts and air is pulled into the chest cavity. When we breathe out, we expel carbon dioxide and other waste gases back into the atmosphere. But when we are stressed or upset, we tend to use the rib muscles to expand the chest. We breathe more quickly, sucking in shallowly. This is excellent in a crisis as it allows us to obtain the optimum amount of oxygen in the shortest possible time, providing our bodies with the extra power needed to handle the emergency. Some people do tend to get stuck in chest-breathing mode, however. Long-term shallow breathing is not only detrimental to physical and emotional health, it can also lead to hyperventilation, panic attacks, chest pains, dizziness and gastro-intestinal problems.

To test your breathing, ask yourself:

- How fast am I breathing as I am reading this?
- Am I pausing between breaths?
- Am I breathing with my chest or with my diaphragm?

A breathing exercise

Start by carrying out instructions 1–6 as given for 'awareness medita-tion' on pages 28–9, with the exception that your eyes should now be closed. Follow the remaining instructions below:

1 Gradually slow down your breathing, inhaling and exhaling as evenly as possible.
2 Place one hand on your chest and the other on your abdomen, just below your rib-cage.
3 As you inhale, allow your abdomen to swell upward. (Your chest should barely move.)
4 As you exhale, let your abdomen flatten.

Give yourself a few minutes to get into a smooth, easy rhythm. As worries and distractions arise, don't hang on to them. Wait calmly for them to float out of your mind – then focus once more on your breathing.

When you feel ready to end the exercise, open your eyes. Allow yourself time to become alert before getting up. With practice, you will begin breathing with your diaphragm quite naturally – and in times of stress, you should be able to correct your breathing without too much effort.

Finding other ways to fill your rest periods

If you have severe or very severe CFS/ME you may need to spend several hours in bed during the day, at least during the early stages of your recovery protocol. This time can be filled, to some extent, with awareness meditation and use of the deep breathing relaxation technique, as described earlier in this chapter. However, this may still leave you with a few hours to fill. Lying in bed with nothing at all to do is massively frustrating and invariably provokes tension, so it is best to find other ways of occupying your rest time.

Audio books

I use pacing to cope with my fibromyalgia and accompanying fatigue, which means that I need to lie in or on my bed between activity sessions for a total of around six hours during the day. I do watch daytime TV for two or three hours, I must admit, but find I can relax better by listening to audio books (also known as 'talking books'). These are available on cassette and CD from most libraries, internet auction sites and internet bookshops, such as <amazon.co.uk>.

Note, though, that audio books are not helpful for everyone. Some people have difficulty concentrating for long spells on the dialogue and others find that the voice in their ears merely sends them to sleep, particularly if the voice has a monotone quality.

Using audio equipment to learn a language or more about an interest

I spend up to half an hour every other day listening to a language cassette or CD, as I am trying to learn Spanish. Learning of any kind uses energy, however, and can keep you from relaxing as much as you need to. For that reason, I don't recommend using audio equipment to learn a language or more about an interest when you feel very tired already. However, if you do feel up to learning in this way for a short while, it will give you the feeling that you've made good use of your time.

Listening to radio podcasts

Downloading radio podcasts from the internet on to an iPod or MP3 player is another good option for filling your time. On the BBC website alone, podcasts are available on many different subjects, including arts and drama, comedy and quizzes, entertainment, factual, history, news and current affairs, health and medical matters, science, soap and sport. The website address is <www.bbc.co.uk/radio/podcasts>.

I spend a great deal of my 'down-time' listening to radio podcasts. Here there are no distracting announcements or commercials as you would find on some radio stations, and the very best of the broadcast is selected from what was originally aired. For me, the comedy and entertainment podcasts are excellent – they frequently make me laugh out loud, which is a tonic in itself. I find I can concentrate without effort when I am being entertained, and I feel 'lifted' afterwards.

It's best to listen to the more serious subjects when you feel in the mood – but only choose subjects that interest you. For example, I like listening to history, medical and science programmes, and again the best of the original broadcast is selected for the podcast. If I do find it difficult to concentrate on the subject matter, I simply skip to the next podcast.

If you don't own a computer, it's likely that someone in your family or a friend does. Podcasts are renewed every few days, so there are always plenty to choose from. However, this may also mean that you need to ask the person who owns the computer if he or she will very kindly download for you on a regular basis.

Listening to music

Another option for your down-time is listening to some of your favourite music. From my own experience, listening to my fairly limited range of CDs became boring after a while – mainly because I was ending up listening to the same tunes over and over as I couldn't afford to keep buying new CDs. To enable you to listen to a wide range of music (of your choice), having a computer comes in handy once again. It enables you to download a vast quantity on to an iPod or MP3 player, and you can shuffle your selection to make it more interesting.

If you don't own a computer, iPod or MP3 player, I would suggest that you ask for an MP3 player for your birthday or Christmas – they're fairly inexpensive and tiny enough to take with you when you need to lie down in other people's houses, and so on. If you don't own a computer, you will again need to ask someone in your family or circle of friends to kindly download a good amount of your favourite music for you. In this instance, one download of a large variety of tunes should last you for months.

Watching TV, videos and DVDs

If you need to spend several hours at a time resting in bed, you may find that listening to audio books, radio broadcasts, music and so on starts to have the opposite effect from that intended – it can get on your nerves. For me, it's the constant noise in my ears that eventually irritates, even though I have the volume fairly low, so I switch off and use the awareness meditation technique for 15–20 minutes to help me unwind. I then choose to watch something on TV, a video, a DVD or internet TV. Watching a film or programme that you find interesting and easy to follow can be very relaxing. However, as with any form of entertainment where you are required to be static, visual performances can become boring and may start to wind you up after a time. Spending several hours at a time watching TV and so on may even leave you with the feeling that you've wasted your day.

Variety helps

It is best to indulge in a *variety* of pastimes during your rest periods – to 'mix it up', as it were. What exactly you choose to do depends, of course, on your particular likes and dislikes, as well as your ability to concentrate at a particular time. Because you are likely to be more alert and receptive in the morning, it is recommended that you try to learn something (by means of audio equipment) at that time of day – that's if you want to learn something and have enough mental stamina to focus your mind for up to half an hour.

Below is an example of how a person with CFS/ME may wish to break up his or her down-time. How you break up your own down-time depends, of course, on how much rest you really need to take and how much of that time you are able to concentrate on learning.

7.30–10.00	*up and about*
10.00–10.15	learning a language/listening to a 'science news' podcast
10.15–11.00	listening to a comedy or entertainment podcast
11.00–11.30	watching TV
11.30–13.30	*up and about*
13.30–14.00	awareness meditation
14.00–14.30	listening to music
14.30–15.00	listening to an audio book
15.00–16.30	*up and about*
16.30–17.00	relaxation exercise
17.00–17.30	listening to a comedy or entertainment podcast
17.30–18.30	watching TV
18.30–19.30	*up and about*
19.30–21.30	watching a DVD (with your partner, relative or friend)
21.30–22.30	*up and about*
22.30	listening to calming music for half an hour before attempting to go to sleep

Sitting-up rest periods

If you don't need to spend time in bed during the day and are able to rest sitting down, that's great! Instead of collapsing in front of the TV for several hours, you may be able to spend some of the time writing, reading or doing something enjoyable at the computer. You may even be able to carry out a hobby such as card-making or writing poetry. However, don't be tempted to overdo it, and don't forget to incorporate awareness meditation and a relaxation exercise into your day.

Sleep problems and CFS/ME

Getting a good night's sleep is of great importance to every human being on the planet. It helps to restore our energy, gives our joints and soft tissues a chance to rest and helps us to cope with stress and problems arising in daily life. Unfortunately, however, for people with CFS/ME – the very ones who most need good restorative sleep – a good night's sleep can be most elusive. Research has found that the fatigue, muscular aches and pains, concentration problems and so on of people with CFS/ME are usually a product of the processes which cause disturbed sleep. The result is poorer and poorer sleep accompanied by a gradual decline into increasing fatigue and other symptoms.

The normal sleep process

Stage 1 of the normal sleep process is the transition from wakefulness through to drowsiness and then light sleep, known as alpha-wave sleep. During this time, sensory awareness gradually lessens until we slide into sound sleep – this is Stage 2 of the process, known as beta-wave sleep. When awakened during Stage 2, we often deny being asleep. Stages 3 and 4 (gamma- and delta-wave sleep) are the deepest stages of sleep. If awakened during either of these stages, we tend to be groggy and temporarily confused.

Stages 1–2 are also known as non-rapid eye movement sleep, as the rapid eye movements (REM) that occur when we dream are absent. REM sleep, during which we dream, can occur at any point in Stages 3 and 4 and usually lasts between 20 and 30 minutes. However, the entire cycle from Stage 1 through to REM sleep takes only about 90 minutes to complete. In one night, it is normal to experience approximately five 90-minute cycles, with the lighter stages of sleep becoming far shorter as the night goes on.

Sleep problems in CFS/ME

Despite spending many hours in bed at night, it is common for people with CFS/ME to wake up tired and feeling as if they have hardly slept at all. The main reason for this appears to be that the deeper stages of sleep – i.e. gamma- and delta-wave sleep – are constantly interrupted by alpha-wave periods of lighter sleep, as has been shown in a range of studies. Being deprived of deep sleep in this way depletes energy levels further, causes irritability and can severely impair both mental and physical performance during the long day ahead. A return to better sleep is therefore essential to improvement.

Getting better sleep

The following suggestions can help you to get better quality sleep:

- As caffeine is a stimulant, reduce the daily amount of caffeine you consume in coffee, tea, cola drinks and chocolate. It is best not to take caffeine at all in the three or four hours before bedtime.
- Avoid eating for at least two hours before bedtime.
- If possible, use the bed and bedroom only for sleeping (and sex). Of course, this may not be possible if your condition dictates that you rest on your bed during daylight hours.
- Ensure that the bedroom heating is not too high. A cooler bedroom is more conducive to sleep.
- As sleeping and waking times tend to be erratic in CFS/ME, try to go to bed at the same time every night. Routine is the best way to regulate your body clock. The recommended amount of sleep is seven to eight hours per night for adults, so try not to sleep longer than this.
- A quiet period before bedtime helps you to feel calm and prepares you for sleep. For example, instead of watching a late-night action film, try reading a book (something gentle, not a rip-roaring thriller) or listening to calming music.
- Have a warm bath, followed by a warm milky drink, before going to bed.
- Don't watch TV in the bedroom before trying to sleep. If you need a TV in the bedroom for entertainment during time in bed during the day, don't turn it on in the hour or so before you want to go to sleep.
- Turn your bedside clock around so you are not tempted to keep checking the time.
- If you can't prevent certain thoughts or ideas running around your

mind, get up for a few minutes and write them down – you are then more likely to stop thinking about them.

- If sleep evades you, try counting down from 301. If you forget which number you're on, just continue from the last number you remember. As this strategy doesn't work for everyone, don't persevere if it isn't working for you.

- When you just can't get to sleep, don't start tossing and turning. Instead, get up, make yourself a warm milky drink and for half an hour try reading a book you find boring. For such occasions, perhaps you could keep a book on a subject that doesn't hold any particular interest for you – a recipe book, an encyclopaedia, a list of research results or instructions for using certain household items.

- If you think that the medication you are taking interferes with your sleep, tell your doctor. There is likely to be an alternative that can be prescribed for you.

- If you can't get enough sleep no matter what you try, ask your doctor to refer you to a sleep therapist.

How to wake up more easily

Some people with CFS/ME find it difficult to wake up in the morning, and then feel muzzy and confused for quite some time afterwards. Fortunately, there are things you can do to help you feel more alert in the morning, as listed below:

- Get up at the same time every morning – this helps to regulate your body clock.

- If you need an alarm to wake you up at a certain time, place it out of reach so you have to get out of bed to turn it off.

- If you don't use an alarm, try to get out of bed as soon as you wake up. The longer you put off getting up, the harder it is.

- Open your curtains before taking your clothes to the bathroom (don't forget to put on your dressing gown first!). Daylight can help you to feel more alert.

Naps

A nap is defined as a short sleep that ends before deep sleep occurs. It comprises of light sleep for a period of less than one hour, and it is taken during the period between getting up and going to bed properly at night. The modern term for a reinvigorating nap is a 'power nap', as coined by James Maas, an American social psychologist. According to studies, a 20-minute nap in the afternoon is more beneficial than an extra 20 minutes in bed in the morning.

Naps that make you feel invigorated afterwards have the obvious benefits of staving off drowsiness and encouraging improved mental and physical function. It's a fact, though, that naps which make you feel better afterwards have a detrimental longer-term effect, as discussed below. In reality, many people with CFS/ME find naps unrefreshing – even draining – yet they can't seem to stop taking them. Indeed, they see naps as evil traps that suck out any remaining energy. Waking from a nap feeling more tired than you did beforehand can also lead to feelings of self-doubt and concerns that you are simply lazy and don't need to nap at all. It's important to remember that people with CFS/ME are in no way lazy. They can easily fall into the habit of resting more than they really need to, but this is understandable as it's due to an intense fear of the effects of fatigue.

There are three general sleep patterns in CFS/ME:

- *Refreshing naps and sleep* – Some people feel very sleepy for a lot of the time, and it seems they can only get through the day if they take regular naps. They sleep well at night, too. If this sounds like you, you may think there's no real harm in continuing the pattern, but you may be surprised to learn that napping is likely to be a part of your fatigue problem. It is therefore recommended that you gradually take fewer naps and shorten their length. As a result, your stamina levels should improve and your fatigue should be reduced.
- *Refreshing naps and unrefreshing sleep* – Some people take several reinvigorating naps during the day but then sleep badly at night. Obviously, reducing the quantity of such naps will encourage more refreshing night-time sleep, with all the benefits that brings.
- *Generalized sleep* – Some people are able to function reasonably well so long as they sleep for about two hours during the day (such a long sleep will normally involve 'deep sleep' and cannot be termed a 'nap'). They also sleep for 12–14 hours during the night. When such people can cut down the lengths of their night and daytime sleeping, they find themselves able to function far better.

How to cut down on napping

Whether your naps and night-time sleep are refreshing or not, you can improve your condition by taking fewer naps. It may have become a habit to fall asleep when resting, particularly if you are lying in a comfortable bed, so the pattern needs to be broken. Here are some ideas to help you stay awake:

- If you prefer lying in the bed rather than on a sofa, try lying on top of the bed-covers rather than between the sheets. You can then cover yourself with a patterned throw or blanket – something that reminds you more of a picnic than sleep.
- Alternate your rest pastimes (such as listening to audio books or music and watching TV) fairly often, before you start to drift into sleep out of boredom.
- Make a phone call to a good friend or favourite family member while lying down, perhaps using a hands-free phone or headset. Reconnecting with people you care about can be a great relaxation tool; it also stops you from falling asleep. Official phone calls and calls to more difficult people can be quite stressful so are best carried out during your up-and-about time rather than in your rest periods.
- Only go to bed at night when you feel tired. Organize your pacing chart to ensure that you are up and about (having a warm milky drink followed by a bath, perhaps) before finally retiring at night.
- Get into the habit of rising at the same time every morning.
- If you normally have a long sleep after lunch, plan your activity chart so that you take a walk outdoors for at least some of that time. Exercise aids digestion and has the effect of making you feel more 'awake'.
- If, as the weeks pass, you are having a real struggle to stay awake while lying down, try setting an alarm for every 20 minutes. At first this may make you feel edgy or even angry – being woken as soon as you fall asleep is far from pleasant. However, the anticipation of being so rudely woken should stop you falling asleep, enabling you to turn off the alarm just before it rings. Going to bed at night should feel very different – the room is now dark and you know that you can sleep undisturbed. Indeed, you may find yourself sleeping better than you did previously at night, thanks to the relief of knowing the alarm won't go off, at least until morning.

Insomnia

Good sleep is essential for survival. When we sleep properly at night, every part of our bodies goes through a vital regeneration process and our muscles and soft tissues are able to thoroughly relax. With good sleep, we wake up feeling refreshed and ready to face the day. It isn't always this way, however – especially for someone with CFS/ME. One symptom of the condition is difficulty getting enough sleep at night (insomnia), a problem that is often made worse by taking daytime naps, as discussed in the previous few pages. The problem is also caused by the abnormal brain wave patterns found in some people with CFS/ME, and this makes it very difficult to achieve deep, restorative sleep.

The insomnia often linked with CFS/ME is defined as the chronic inability to fall asleep or experience uninterrupted sleep, and it can follow any of the patterns listed below. You may have periods of time where your body sticks to one particular pattern, then periods when it sticks to another. It is also possible for your sleep pattern to be different virtually every night.

- You can't get to sleep for two or three hours after going to bed.
- You go to sleep easily enough, but wake up in the early hours and have great difficulty going back to sleep.
- You wake up several times during the night, sometimes for short periods and sometimes for longer periods.
- You wake too early in the morning and can't get back to sleep.

Strategies for curing insomnia

There are several other 'natural' strategies for encouraging a return to a good sleeping rhythm, but it might be an idea to also use tricyclic medication for up to three months. This will provide added help for getting a good night's sleep.

Develop good sleep habits by doing the following (some of these suggestions have already been mentioned in this chapter):

- Take fewer naps, and sleep for a shorter duration – no longer than half an hour. All naps, even those that are not energizing, can prevent you from feeling sleepy at bedtime.
- Hang heavy curtains to make the bedroom as dark as possible.
- Before trying to sleep, unwind by listening to music or a relaxation tape, reading or watching an unexciting programme on TV.
- Have a warm drink.
- Shortly before bedtime take a warm bath (preferably using relaxing aromatherapy oils, as discussed on page 97).
- Go to bed when you feel sleepy, so long as it is not before 9.30 p.m.
- Ensure that your bed and bedroom are comfortably warm, but not over-heated.
- Wear a sleep mask to help you sleep soundly for longer periods of time.
- Wear earplugs to eliminate distracting noises.
- Make yourself comfortable in bed, breathing slowly and evenly into your diaphragm. Clear your mind and allow your thoughts to drift. Don't hold on to any one thought, but let them pass unchecked.
- Set your alarm for the same time every morning.

Try to avoid the following:

- caffeine drinks after 6 p.m.;
- alcohol before bedtime;
- eating, drinking or reading in bed;
- engaging in animated conversation (or arguments) before bedtime;
- napping during the day;
- sitting up to watch TV for long periods, particularly in the evening.

Taking up the last point: sitting to watch TV for several hours during daytime and evening is a habit that not only causes stiffness and muscle pain, it also interferes with sleep. This is because TV provokes numerous emotional responses in rapid succession, quickening the heart-rate and releasing chemicals (such as adrenaline) for no useful purpose. When these chemicals are produced naturally, we deal with the situation and our bloodflow is returned to normal. However, when chemicals are induced second-hand – such as occurs when watching TV – they remain in the bloodstream. This causes tension to linger, and ultimately gives rise to more muscle pains.

Additional tips to encourage better sleep

Here are a few more tips to improve your sleep:

- Pace yourself according to the dictates of your pacing chart, only adding extra activities and reducing rest time when you are stable and feel up to doing so.
- Learn to say 'no', so that you don't push yourself unnecessarily.
- Try to do something you enjoy every day.
- If possible, take a daily stroll – it doesn't have to be a long one. A short walk is better than no walk at all.
- If you go to work in the morning, get up 15 minutes earlier than usual so you are not tempted to rush around.
- Eat a low-calorie, high-fibre breakfast such as grapefruit followed by porridge oats, or breakfast cereal followed by wholemeal toast. Avoid sugary cereals.
- Drink natural fruit juice at breakfast – not juices with added sugar or sweeteners. Alternatively, drink warm boiled water with freshly squeezed lemon juice.
- Eat something every three or four hours and don't skip meals.
- As eating a very low-calorie diet has the effect of increasing fatigue, don't try to count calories.
- If you are following a daily exercise routine, try to avoid doing this in the six hours before bedtime.

Wakefulness due to anxiety

People who have difficulty falling asleep at night are known to be more likely than others to focus on problems, worries and any noises around them, especially if they don't fall asleep straight away. If this is the case with you, you should find that using cognitive behavioural therapy, as discussed in Chapter 4, can make you less anxious. The recommendations on page 40 can also be a great help. If all else fails, you may need to be prescribed either an anti-anxiety medication or a tricyclic antidepressant (see below), at least for the short term. Speak to your doctor if you think you need this kind of help.

Sleep medications

The insomnia of CFS/ME can be improved by taking a tricyclic antidepressant medication such as imipramine, amitriptyline, doxepin, trazodone or lofepramine. Tricyclic antidepressants are available from your doctor on prescription and work by increasing the concentration of chemicals that are known to promote sleep, reducing pain levels and easing muscle tension – you don't need to be depressed to take them. To prevent the feeling of a 'thick head' the next morning, tricyclics are best taken in the evening rather than immediately before bedtime. The possible side-effects include foggy brain, weight gain, constipation, dizziness, nausea, sweating, dry mouth and short-term memory problems.

Over-the-counter sleep medications can increase the duration of sleep but will not lengthen deep sleep, which is essential for tissue repair and regeneration of tissues. Tricyclic antidepressants, however, can encourage deep sleep. If you have been prescribed this kind of medication but it is no longer effective, the dosage may need adjusting or you may need to try another type.

Vitamin D3

It's possible to take a simple laboratory test to find out whether you have a deficiency of vitamin D3 – a hormone that is integral to the sleep process. It is best taken in liquid form and placed by a dropper on to the tongue before going to bed – 4000 IU, taken in two 2000 IU drops, seems to work best. If you are interested in this option, speak to your doctor.

5-HTP (hydroxy-tryptophan)

When vitamin D3 is taken in combination with a chemical called 5-HTP – which raises levels of a sleep-inducing chemical in the body called serotonin – sleep patterns can revert to normal within a few days. It is recommended that 100–200 mg of 5-HTP is taken daily with vitamin D3 until lab tests show that you are no longer deficient of the vitamin.

If you are suffering from depression as well as sleeplessness, you can take 100 mg dosages of 5-HTP three or four times daily without the need for lab tests beforehand. Depression often responds well to a return to the normal sleep rhythm, adrenal gland support (which 5-HTP offers) and vitamin and mineral therapy, as discussed in Chapter 5.

4

Emotional support

People with CFS/ME must live their lives in the face of overwhelming fatigue, which obviously causes considerable distress. The result is often chronic anxiety, negative thinking and the feeling that no one really understands. However, there are techniques which can help you to gradually overcome difficult emotions, as explained in this chapter.

Overcoming difficult emotions

The negative emotions discussed in this section are common in CFS/ME.

Feelings of vulnerability

Vulnerability is a natural human condition. We all need people to love us; we all crave the affirmation of others. To a large extent we are all dependent upon others, measuring their responses to reassure ourselves that we are worthwhile human beings, that we are indeed loveable. When we are chronically ill, as well as feeling unattractive we believe we have little to offer the people around us – therefore we fear we are no longer loveable.

Feelings of vulnerability will always be present in chronic illness, but it is possible to defeat the worst of them by looking less to outsiders for affirmation. We all have inner strengths and particular talents, and we may be unaware of many of these. Yet if we waited for others to point them out we would probably be waiting for ever!

Your particular forte may be in planning and organizing, or problem solving, or handling finances – not necessarily out of the family setting. You may be an authority on steam engines, a good cook, a great listener, a talented artist, an excellent singer or a competent driver. Please do not underestimate yourself!

Feelings of guilt

It is common to want to blame someone for the fact that you are ill, and many imagine that they themselves must have done something very wrong to deserve such 'punishment'. Blaming either yourself or others is pointless, however. Life is a lottery. Some people are rich, some poor; some are clever, some not so clever; some fall ill, some remain healthy – that's just the way it is.

You may, after learning that improvement lies mainly in your own hands, feel guilty for making no tangible progress. Assuming you have at least tried to help yourself, it's important to remember that there is probably a sound reason for your failure. For example, you may have been unable to find information about exactly how to help yourself; you may be held back by additional health problems; or you may not have allowed sufficient time for any improvements to show.

Increased fatigue and other symptoms are a constant threat in CFS/ME, and they often result from outside influences such as the weather, a fall or a family crisis. It may, however, have been an activity you chose to do that caused the exacerbation – and so you feel guilty. Viewing a symptom increase as a learning experience may be of some consolation – for instance, you attempted to bake a cake, but afterwards you were exhausted and felt ill. Although it was a hard lesson, you learned that you are not yet ready to do any baking.

Guilt may also arise if you think you are a burden on your family. Maybe you feel bad about their extra workload and the fact that their free time is now so limited. When a person with CFS/ME needs a full-time carer, it is important that the carer has time to him- or herself, retains certain interests and has occasional 'time off'. Knowing that your carer is enjoying life regardless of your ill-health and limitations – which of course he or she has a perfect right to do – should help you to feel less guilty.

Feelings of fear

When you have an illness for which there is, as yet, no absolute cure, it is natural to worry about the future. It's also natural to be afraid of deteriorating further, of becoming entirely dependent upon others and of the long-term effects of medication. Unfortunately, chronic illness exerts profound effects on the individual. It is not always easy to be cheerful and bright when you have a cold, never mind an energy-sapping illness to which you can see no end. At least you know that a cold will soon pass; at least you can tell yourself that your spirits will then be restored. People with CFS/ME know nothing of the sort.

However, in most cases of CFS/ME, the fear of the unknown abates with time. You learn that you can take pleasure from family life, you can enjoy social occasions, you can take up interests and hobbies, and you can be of use to others. Most important, you learn that your condition really can improve and that your future looks far less grim than you once thought.

Feelings of uselessness

When tasks that were once accomplished with ease have now either to be performed in stages or dropped altogether, you can feel pretty useless. It is the same with many of your enjoyable activities – and not necessarily ones requiring much effort. Indeed, even activities requiring mental focus such as reading or writing can be exhausting for someone with CFS/ME. Don't give up hope of ever again being able to do the things you enjoyed, however. The heaviest and most taxing of activities may be permanently out of your scope, but other pleasures (and tasks) can be achieved, given time, patience and the employment of pain and stress management strategies, as discussed later in this chapter.

Cognitive behavioural therapy

Because unhealthy ways of thinking and behaving can hinder the recovery process, a treatment known as cognitive behavioural therapy (CBT, for short) is highly recommended. CBT uses a set of structured psychological techniques to tackle negative thought patterns, and is very useful when used in combination with a gradual increase in activity levels and therapies such as diet, exercise and stress management techniques. Indeed, when researchers assessed data from 15 studies into the effects of CBT on 1,043 CFS/ME patients, they concluded that CBT is far more effective than older conventional treatments at reducing symptom severity.

Your doctor should be able to refer you to a CBT therapist who will identify how you are thinking and in what ways this is hampering your recovery. The therapy is normally performed in up to 20 hour-long sessions.

Many CBT techniques are incorporated in the advice in this chapter, too.

Coping with other people

Most people are spurred into activity at the sight of, say, a traffic accident. Instinctively forming a team, 'onlookers' each play a part in trying to help the injured – making them as comfortable as possible, warning and diverting approaching traffic and alerting the emergency services. In some instances, onlookers go so far as to put their own lives at risk in their determination to help a person – or even an animal – in trouble. However, those same people are rarely galvanized into action when the crisis is not obvious, for example when someone suffering from an invisible illness such as CFS/ME complains of feeling exhausted.

Why do people distrust what I say?

Sadly, it's human nature to be suspicious, which means that some people tag CFS/ME sufferers as soft and attention-seeking. Being judged in this way is greatly upsetting, especially as the reverse is true in most cases – experts now believe that the majority of people with CFS/ME play down their symptoms as the result of past derision from others. As a result, they may get into the habit of muttering, 'I'm not too bad, thanks,' or 'A bit better today ...' Unfortunately, however, playing down a little-understood condition such as CFS/ME can actually come across as indecision about whether you are feeling ill at all! Moreover, vague, half-hearted responses only serve to water any seeds of doubt in the other person's mind.

It's a fact that conveying to others the nature, severity and complexity of CFS/ME is, without doubt, slavishly hard work. The key is to be straightforward, open and brief – listeners get bored when people 'harp on' about their ill-health. But if you don't at least try to explain, certain people around you may never understand

Standing up for yourself

Because sarcastic and derisory remarks from others can chip away at your confidence, they should not pass unchallenged. Standing up for yourself is not easy, but doing so can have a releasing effect. Failing to stand up for yourself, on the other hand, usually leaves you feeling hurt, offended and very resentful. You are also likely to feel angry with yourself for allowing yourself to be hurt.

If your partner were to complain, 'I do all the housework while you do absolutely nothing,' it is suggested that you respond: 'I'm trying as hard as I can, but nearly everything I do makes me feel worse. I know it seems unfair when you're stuck with all the housework, so maybe it will help you to know that seeing you so busy is not easy for me. I really do appreciate your efforts, though. Perhaps we should try to put up with a bit of dust and clutter?' If the initial comment was made during a heated exchange, you could answer, 'That's a hurtful thing to say. I may be doing very little, but it's not my fault. I'd like to talk this through when we're calmer.'

If family members are sceptical of your condition, no matter what words or manner you employ, you may be so hurt you consider cutting yourself off from them completely. This is perhaps your best option if they condemn you relentlessly, but not otherwise. Indeed, occasional scepticism and ill-judged remarks are best tackled by keeping on steadily stating your case, remembering to bring all unfair comments to their attention.

It may help you to know that when someone close to you remains deaf to your assertions of fatigue and so on, it is often because they can't face the fact that a person they love is experiencing chronic ill-health. The only way they know how to deal with your illness is to refuse to believe in it. In effect, they cope by not coping, which is actually their problem, not yours. Don't ever give up on them, though, for viewpoints often change with time.

It may be that people outside your immediate circle of friends and relatives make derisory comments – but they have no right to hurt you, and should not get away with it. Your best weapons here are words that make them think. For example, a person who asks mockingly, 'Are we any better today?' could be met with, 'Is there something on your mind? If so, just say it … If you really are concerned about my health, thank you. The truth is I'm feeling worn out and don't know how I'll manage to get home.'

CFS/ME and your friends

As you may already have discovered, having CFS/ME leaves you in little doubt as to who your real friends are. The 'friends' who are offended when you back out of a planned get-together, the 'friends' who are unconvinced when you explain that, yes, you were able to have a night out with them last week but you feel too ill to go out tonight, and the 'friends' who complain that you have let them down again are really not worth your precious energies. Their negative input into your life is detrimental to your confidence as well as to your health.

Guilt is a natural consequence of letting people down. The feeling is amplified when you have to renege on prearranged activities on a regular basis. Knowing it causes ill-feeling in certain people may spur you into attempting activities you know will make you suffer, and you may turn up at the next social event despite feeling particularly wiped out and despite knowing that doing so is likely to provoke a flare-up of symptoms. Is placing yourself at risk in this way really worth the fact that you have temporarily assuaged your guilt? I think not.

What about the 'friends' who, after you have been unable to socialize as before, have gradually dropped out of your life? Can you honestly say they were true friends? Wouldn't a true friend make allowances for your illness? Wouldn't a true friend try to understand what

you were going through? Yes, CFS/ME certainly allows you to differen-
tiate between true friends and fair-weather friends.

Why do people make me feel so upset?

Even if everyone was charming and accepting around you, CFS/ME
would be a frustrating, upsetting, anger-making business. We all know
the condemnation experienced by someone who is frequently off sick
from work. Before you became ill, you may even have thought badly of
someone who regularly complained of ill-health. We know that society
in general is contemptuous of both mental and physical weakness.
When we become ill, all this knowledge seems to form a tight ball in
our heads. It only takes one careless comment and we either explode
into rage or feel so upset and despairing we want to hide ourselves
away.

Without doubt, some people are incredibly insensitive. You may
feel you are always on your guard, dreading the remark that will send
you into a whirl of anger or spiralling into the depths of despair. Sadly,
chronic invisible illness lays the individual wide open to the precon-
ceptions of others. As I mentioned earlier, hurtful comments should
never pass unchallenged. If the perpetrator appears contrite, go on to
briefly explain just how the illness affects you.

Negative thinking

A lot of our negative thinking arises from early conditioning. Indeed,
the children of parents who consistently make the same type of
comment often grow up with similar basic attitudes. For example, if
a woman regularly scoffs at weakness, or if her husband repeatedly
declares that incompetence is unforgivable, their children have a fair
chance of growing up believing this way of thinking is valid and proper.

When people frequently voice negative thoughts, it generally means
they are afraid of the very thing about which they are being negative.
The mother mentioned above, who decries weakness in others, does so
because she secretly fears she is weak, and the father who denounces
incompetence in others does so because he has deep-seated fears
about his own competence. When their children copy these attitudes
into adulthood, condemning weakness and incompetence as well as
displaying other negative viewpoints, this, too, stems from inherent
beliefs that they are lacking in many ways.

Approaching life's ups and downs with a particular mindset – such as
trust or distrust, enthusiasm or depression, self-assurance or timidity – is
usually due to childhood conditioning. Our automatic thoughts are,
therefore, determined by whatever mindsets are built into our char-

acters, controlling our behaviour in any given situation. For example, when planning a birthday party, a person with a depressive mindset will dread the 'big day', worrying that few guests will turn up. A person with an enthusiastic mindset, on the other hand, will eagerly await the party, certain of its success. A person with a trustful mindset will take, 'That sweater's a bit small for you, love,' as a caring remark and happily change into something more 'fitting', whereas a person with a distrustful mindset will take it as a criticism of his or her weight, of the sweater, of his or her choice of attire, or of all these things put together!

Irrational feelings

People with negative mindsets invariably have irrational feelings about themselves, and these feelings often become self-fulfilling prophesies. For example, 'I will never be any good with money' stops you trying to be good with money, 'I will never make anyone happy' stops you trying to make anyone happy and, concerning your ill-health, 'I am no fun to have around any more' makes you stop trying to retain a good-humoured attitude. These irrational feelings are untruths that unfortunately determine the person's behaviour, and chronic illness is often the spark that sets irrational feelings blazing out of control.

With training in CBT techniques, irrational thoughts and feelings can be turned around, and it's possible to learn a new, more positive approach to life. First, however, it is necessary to acknowledge irrational thoughts and feelings for what they are, and for the behaviour they induce. Up-coming family celebrations commonly provoke feelings of anxiety in people with CFS/ME. Actually writing down your thoughts and feelings, and really analysing them, can make the fact that they are irrational crystal clear. It makes you more aware.

Here is an example of possible irrational thoughts and feelings prior to a family party:

Situation	Irrational thoughts	Irrational feelings
Family party	I will be a real wet blanket. No one will want to talk to me. I will put a dampener on the whole event.	I will then feel sad, hurt and alienated. I will hate myself for being such a misery.

This example illustrates just how irrational chronic illness can sometimes make you. Yet without analysis, the potential repercussions can be staggering. In this situation, you may end up talking yourself into staying at home, experiencing mixed self-pity, guilt and even self-loathing. Your decision could even cause an argument with your partner.

The example also reveals a common tendency for people to worry about something which may never happen. If you are feeling terrible already, don't fret about a family party scheduled for the weekend! You are hardly likely to be well enough to attend – and your family should be made aware of that fact. However, if you are no worse than usual, then, realistically, staying at home is not the answer. No matter how dire your 'normal' condition, you need, for the sake of your sanity, to have a life; you need to be with others occasionally – therefore you need to make an extra effort every now and again. Given sufficient forward planning, certain events really can be managed effectively, for whether your symptoms are severe or not, backing out of events/activities you may otherwise have enjoyed can leave you feeling angry at yourself, furious with your illness, and resentful that everyone else is in good health. (See pages 20–21 for more information on coping with special occasions.)

My own CBT therapist taught me to record my thoughts and feelings prior to a troublesome event, and doing so always helps me. Assuming, then, that you are no worse than usual, try to write down your expectations of what will happen at the party, as described above. Now look objectively at what you have written. Are your thoughts and feelings reasonable? Certainly you would feel like a wet blanket if you sat with a face as long as a fiddle and made no effort to talk to anyone! And could you indeed be so rude as to avoid conversing? Are your relatives really so antisocial they would disregard you?

When we challenge negative feelings thus, the reality of the situation soon becomes apparent. People make an effort to be friendly at family gatherings. Your fellow guests are people you know well. Common ground can always be found, should you wish to look for it.

So, you have re-evaluated and subsequently vanquished one set of negative thoughts, only to find it is swiftly replaced by another. You have decided to attend the party, but now you are worrying about coping with your fatigue and other symptoms in company. Will the exhaustion totally consume you? Will you burst into tears? Will everyone think you pathetic?

It's normal to worry about coping with ill-health of any kind when out of your usual environment, but as a result of your fears your worries may be somewhat distorted. Writing them down helps you see them in a more detached light.

Here is the same example, but this time I have incorporated a column listing possible solutions:

Situation	Irrational thoughts	Irrational feelings	Solution
I will feel wiped out at the party.	I will be unable to cope with the fatigue and muscle aches.	People will think me weak and stupid.	Rest well before attending the party.
I will feel as if I could cry.	They will all hate me for spoiling the occasion.	I will get angry and accuse everyone of not caring. I will then feel angry with myself.	Take painkillers before I leave. Ask to lie down before I start to feel over-tired.

Here, irrational feelings are seen for what they are, and possible solutions are considered – you may even want to ask your hosts beforehand if you could please lie down in a warm room after a while, or prepare them for your early departure. Looking for realistic ways to help you through a certain situation is far more useful than immersing yourself in worries which get you nowhere. More importantly, it can help you to cope with some degree of fatigue.

You may then find yourself assailed by further worries. You have planned to ask if you might lie down, but when the time comes feel anxious about actually doing so. Surely your hosts will think you feeble and demanding! Surely everyone will stare and whisper behind your back! This again is irrational thinking, and since obviously you won't always be able to write down your feelings, you should mentally consider what you need to do. In this instance, all you can do, unless you want to risk an increase in symptoms as well as thoughts of self-loathing, is ask.

From personal experience, I can honestly say that people are only too willing to assist when asked directly. It often happens that they aren't really sure what to say or how to help you, so when you ask for help of a particular kind it takes the pressure off them. They will probably then want to know whether the bedroom is warm enough, the mattress firm enough, the pillows soft enough ... If they do scowl and make a comment to the effect that you are making a fuss – and in all my years of asking others for help (there is a large fatigue component to my fibromyalgia) I have never come across anyone who has – it says a lot more about their nature than yours!

Helping others to understand

In attempting to help the people you care about understand your health problems, you should try to speak clearly and openly. Brevity also has a positive impact, as has being honest about how you feel.

Speaking openly

Before endeavouring to describe your feelings, you first need to focus on how you actually do feel. It may be difficult to admit you feel guilty, frustrated, angry, useless, vulnerable and so on, even to yourself. Sharing your feelings with others is even more difficult, yet it is an important step towards halting the problems those feelings can cause. I'll just add that in your need to be understood by others, you should try not to make assumptions about how they feel about you.

Speaking to others in the following way is sure to cause offence: 'I get upset when you think I'm exaggerating!' or 'I don't believe you really care about me, and that makes me feel hopeless!' or 'I'm losing confidence because you treat me as if I'm not trying to help myself!' Such comments are likely to be seen as accusations and may even provoke a quarrel. It is best to speak openly about something that's troubling you, but without implying that the other person is contributing to the problem. This will encourage him or her to take your comments more seriously and even to be more thoughtful. Before you do speak openly of your feelings, however, the following list of considerations should be taken into account:

- *Ensure you have interpreted the other person's behaviour correctly* – For example, you may view your mother bringing you a basket of fruit and vegetables as a criticism of your diet, when in truth it is a goodwill gesture, just to show she cares! You have a perfect right to interpret the words or actions of others in whatever way you wish, but that interpretation is not necessarily reality. In fact, it is amazing how wrong we often are in our perceptions of what others think and feel.

- *Ensure you are specific in recalling another person's behaviour* – For example, 'You never understand how exhausted I get' is far more inflammatory than 'You didn't seem to understand yesterday, when I told you how exhausted I felt.'

- *Ensure that what you are about to say is what you really mean* – For example, statements such as 'Everyone thinks you're insensitive' or 'We all think you've got an attitude problem' are, besides being inflammatory, very unfair. We have no way of knowing that 'everyone' is of the same opinion. The use of the depersonalized 'everyone', 'we' or 'us' – often said in the hope of deflecting the listener's anger – can cause more hurt and anger than if the criticism is direct and personal.

It's easy to see how others can misunderstand or take offence when we fail to communicate effectively. Changing the habits of a lifetime is difficult, for it means analysing our thoughts before rearranging them into speech, but we are rewarded for our efforts when people start to listen, when they cease to be annoyed as we carefully explain an area they don't fully understand.

Dealing with co-workers

If you are managing to work and cope with CFS/ME at the same time, well done! Exceptions for chronic ill-health in the workplace generally have to be fought for. Even when your boss is tolerant, your co-workers often are not.

If your CFS/ME is not yet accepted by the people you work with, be prepared for a struggle, and never be tempted to hide any shortcomings related to your health. You need to be able to communicate the nature of your illness and how it affects your performance, otherwise you are liable to be condemned as slow and inefficient, especially by co-workers who may be convinced you are not pulling your weight.

Strangely enough, given sufficient information about your health problems, employers are often more sympathetic than some fellow employees. For example, your exclusion from certain duties can prompt co-workers to make snide remarks out of jealousy and resentment. They may also distrust your claim to illness and so make remarks that are cruel and unjust. Once again, hurtful remarks should not be tolerated!

The thought of objecting to an unfair accusation, particularly when you are at a low ebb, may seem daunting. However, as well as being the only means of getting through to some people, it also helps you maintain self-esteem. For example, a co-worker may remark, 'You're looking fine. I'm sure you're using your so-called illness to get out of doing the filing!' Whether the tone is light or not, the content is hostile and undeserved. Failing to respond – maybe because you are too angry, too hurt or simply too tired – only serves to confirm their opinion. Your answer should be a firm, 'I resent that. I'm glad you think I look okay, but I don't use my illness as an excuse, and I don't have to prove myself to you.' The co-worker will hopefully apologize at this point, and may even confess, 'I suppose I just don't understand what's wrong with you.' Here is your chance to explain further about CFS/ME.

Whenever others appear to be in a receptive frame of mind, grasp the opportunity to explain your condition. Your symptoms may best be understood when you equate them to something within the listener's experience. For instance, 'My symptoms are like having the flu all the time,' helps them see how it is for you. Explain, too, the most troublesome of your additional symptoms, making sure to emphasize that they are all elements of your condition. The more information you can feed to the people around you, the more likely they are to digest it.

Being assertive

If you push yourself beyond your limits in order to please others, it only makes them suppose you are doing what you are capable of doing. Indeed, they will expect the same from you every time. You can avoid this vicious cycle by learning, instead, to please yourself and by speaking up when you need help.

Asking for help is not easy, especially when you have been active and independent all your life. Yet communicating your needs will usually get you what you want. What is the alternative – frustration, anger and a flare-up of symptoms because you have once again overdone it? Asking for help is *not* an indication of weakness or failure, it is a sign of your resolve to face your situation. There is a fine line between being assertive and being demanding, however. Asking for help clearly and politely, then showing gratitude afterwards, creates 'feel-good' emotions in others. It also increases the chances of their offering help in the future.

Learning to say 'no'

Saying 'no' to others is equally difficult – but, for the sake of your health, you need to say it, and as often as necessary. Otherwise, the people in your life will simply assume that you are still able to do most things. For example, if friends 'expect' you to drive 20 miles to see them, it is best to politely explain: 'If I drove all that way, I'd not be up to much else, I'm afraid. It's been a while since we met and I was looking forward to a good chat.' Your friends will probably admit they didn't realize how ill you were and offer to drive to your home instead. However, if they are not satisfied with your reasoning, you should dig in your heels and add, 'The drive home would be a nightmare, as well. To be honest, I'd be so exhausted I wouldn't be safe behind the wheel. I'd be grateful if you could come to see me.' If these people are worthy of the title 'friends', they will now readily agree to your suggestion.

Another example of saying 'no' is if relatives ask you to baby-sit their toddler and you know you are not up to it. In this instance, it is best to say something to the effect of: 'I'd love to look after little Millie, but

I'm just not well enough. What most concerns me is that I wouldn't be able to leap up if she was about to hurt herself.' Wanting the best for their daughter, your family would probably say a hurried, 'Oh, I see. Don't worry, we'll get so-and-so to look after her.'

Don't, under any circumstance, allow anyone to pressure you into doing something you know will provoke an increase in symptoms, and don't put yourself under pressure by feeling obliged to repay someone in kind. Your health is far more important than feelings of duty.

Adjusting your expectations

Thinking about the future is a natural human characteristic. When that future is clouded by the physical and emotional impact of chronic illness, we tend to be plagued by compelling 'what ifs'. It is also common to be haunted by the many bleak and hopeless years we fear are ahead of us.

However, looking ahead with fear is counter-productive. The first step towards conquering this fear is to tell yourself that it does no good. Controlling your thinking is far from easy, but it can be achieved. When the bleak visions loom, try to distract yourself either by turning your mind to something pleasant or, your condition permitting, by doing something that demands concentration. Staving off such visions on a regular basis will gradually become second nature and eventually change your way of thinking.

Living in the present

People with CFS/ME need all their resources to handle the present. This can largely be achieved with the help of the enjoyable yet untaxing leisure interests it is recommended that you find. After all, why sit brooding in your activity periods when you could be reading a gripping book, penning a poem, surfing the internet, taking a walk or sharing views with someone close? This is the time to consider doing things you never had time for before. If, for example, assembling a model railway was a childhood dream you never managed to fulfil, or if you always fancied learning to play the guitar but never quite got around to it, this, CFS/ME permitting, is your opportunity!

Looking on the bright side

Developing a positive outlook is invaluable in CFS/ME. It stops you dwelling on the past, it helps you to enjoy the present, and it bestows hope and conviction. Indeed, looking for something pleasing in the things you do can ease anxiety and stress and so result in improvement.

You may wonder what could possibly be pleasing about washing dishes or peeling potatoes! As most of us perform these tasks by the kitchen window, they have that in their favour. While you scour the pans or peel the spuds, do you consciously appreciate the world outside, or are you inclined to gaze blindly out, fretting about this and that? If the latter is generally the case, concentrate instead on really looking at and appreciating your outdoor environment. For example, try to admire the manifold creations of nature, observe the inventiveness in all that is man-made and notice how people behave as they go about their daily business.

As the seasons pass, consciously appreciate the effects different weather conditions have on your environment. Even the busiest and most depressing of streets can be enhanced by bright sunshine sparkling off wet rooftops, by icicles hanging from window ledges, by a covering of fresh snow. All right, so 'inclement' weather can create numerous problems, but why think of those problems when you're snug and warm indoors? Keep your mind on the present. Let gazing at the weather – the sunshine, the rain, the frost, the snow – stir your senses. Children like to stretch out a hand to feel the rain, they are awed by the sight of icicles and they are excited by snow, yet so often we lose that childish appreciation when we reach adulthood. It's never too late to recapture it, however. The time to worry about harsh weather conditions is shortly before you step outside.

Accepting the things you can't change

Including the weather, there are many things in life we cannot change. We can do nothing about the fact that we are either creative or practical, tall or short, male or female. Neither can we change the fact that we have a chronic illness, although we can certainly improve the situation. Acknowledging the things we can't change – and trying to live with them – is fundamental to stress management.

As well as being distracting, involving yourself in a new challenge can be infinitely rewarding. Consider playing computer games, talking to others with CFS/ME on the internet, taking up model-making, oil-painting, stencilling, playing the keyboard, tapestry-work, glass and china painting, picture-framing, jewellery-making ... the list is endless. The selection of 'things to do' in a craft shop alone is quite dazzling!

Of course, not everyone with CFS/ME is physically able to do such things, especially in the early days of their pacing regime, as discussed in Chapters 1 and 2. These are merely suggestions. The challenge is to find interests which suit your capabilities, as well as ones that stimulate your imagination.

Learning to let go

If CFS/ME forces you to give up your career, you can feel you have lost much of what gave you a sense of worthiness and identity. However, learning to let go of the things you can no longer do, possibly looking to a new, less demanding but equally fulfilling career, and searching out new interests to replace old (more taxing) ones is the only way forward emotionally. People with CFS/ME need to look after their minds as well as their bodies.

If you have had to give up your job, studying part-time at your local college could help you feel less isolated. Whether you fancy acquiring a few academic qualifications or simply taking up a new leisure interest (where the atmosphere is more casual and regular attendance not so important), learning something different can be very rewarding. Studying a subject that is helpful in dealing with your condition – for example, reflexology, aromatherapy, meditation, relaxation, stress management, assertiveness training and so on, may prove invaluable, too.

If you are fairly mobile, aqua aerobics, low-impact aerobics, Pilates or yoga classes can, if you employ caution, help to maintain and ulti-mately improve your strength, stamina and mobility. What's more, they can also provide an outlet for stress. Competitive games – even those of a gentle nature like chess, backgammon, Scrabble and bridge – are not a good idea, for they produce tension and stress.

The people around you

People with CFS/ME desperately need to know that others care. Most of all, they crave the sympathy and understanding of their nearest and dearest, feeling upset when they experience thoughtlessness or impa-tience. Yet sufferers often fail to appreciate that the illness can create huge problems for these very people.

CFS/ME and your partner

It's possible that your partner is more troubled by your ill-health than you realize. He or she can feel guilty for being well and active when you are sick and stagnant; disappointed and confused when you show no sign of recovery; angry and useless for never seeming to be able to say the right thing; and, not least, anxious for his or her own future happiness.

In fact, your partner's concerns are possibly equal to your own. The need for intimacy, companionship and a future to look forward to – mixed with feelings of inadequacy for being unable to ease your suffering – may even prompt doubts about his or her ability to cope indefinitely with a partner who is chronically ill. These misgivings can then be amplified by having to endure reproaches for being insensitive and uncaring.

It is common for a person who is chronically ill to become self-absorbed. The main causes of this are that:

- the physical and emotional drain of dealing with the condition can interfere with your ability to see your partner's viewpoint;
- after experiencing scepticism or indifference from others, you may misinterpret your partner's behaviour.

When a communication breakdown occurs, the relationship can become a battle, with each partner feeling resentful and unloved. Unless each makes an effort to understand the other person, the relationship may flounder. It is a fact that you can only know what your partner is thinking and feeling when you make time to calmly talk problems through. It is certainly worth the effort, for exchanging perceptions, fears and needs carries the bonus of strengthening your relationship.

CFS/ME and other family members

Just as your partner has his or her own needs, so too have other family members. Their needs are basically selfish, as are everyone's. In most cases, their chief need, where you are concerned, is to see you well and smiling again. They won't then have to worry about you so much; they won't be obliged to be so attentive. Once you are 'recovered', you will again be able to accompany them on Saturday shopping trips, to line-dancing class, or to play snooker and squash ... Put simply, you are an important part of their lives, and they want everything 'back to normal'.

As your illness continues, however, their bafflement may turn to irritation. Desperate to see you as you once were, they may prefer to interpret your behaviour as lethargy, self-indulgence or even hypochondria. Remarks such as 'You're not doing anything to help yourself,' or 'You need to get out and enjoy yourself more,' are typical, made in the misguided belief that you need a 'push' to help you back to 'normality'.

Unchecked, such 'advice' can turn to full-scale nagging. Comments such as 'You should try running up and down the stairs twenty times a day – that would improve your stamina,' 'Get out on your bicycle again. It'll do you the power of good,' 'Are you sure you're trying hard enough? Don't you want to get better?' may be delivered repeatedly in a genuine desire to see you fit and well, but they are hurtful and demoralizing. Moreover, when you are told often enough that you are making no effort to improve your condition, you can start to believe it.

Ironically, the people closest to us are the ones most likely to make wounding remarks, which only compounds the hurt. Try to remember, however, that they are the people who are most concerned that you get better. Instead of observing the situation from all angles, they are making the mistake of seeing it through their eyes only.

Leon and Victoria

It is easy to understand why 10-year-old Leon has convinced himself that his mother, Victoria, 39, is not as ill as she says she is. He needs her to make his meals, to run him around in the car, to organize his life ... just to be there, her normal, capable self. He sees her illness as a threat to his whole world. But she looks fine – just the same as ever. In attempting to prove to himself that everything is indeed exactly as it always was, Leon may say, 'You look fine, Mum. Take me to my friend's house tonight, will you?' Victoria explains that she's not up to driving, but Leon bursts out, 'You don't want to do anything for me any more! I don't think you love me!' So, despite the fact that Victoria feels exhausted, has a headache and can barely think straight, she gets into the car and takes her son to see his friend. Consequently, Leon is reassured. Victoria, however, feels more unwell than ever and is upset that her child can't seem to understand.

Leon's demands persist because, in capitulating, Victoria is proving she can still do as much for him as ever. He will only accept her illness if she continually reassures him of her love, yet firmly explains why she cannot be as active as before. When children know where they stand, they soon adapt.

Charlotte, Scott and Freya

Charlotte, 25, is mother to 18-month-old Freya, and has recently been diagnosed with CFS/ME. She makes keeping Freya clean, safe and fed a priority, but she feels a failure for neglecting the housework, annoyed that her husband, Scott, expects home life to be as happy and ordered as it was before she became ill, and cheated for being too ill to really *enjoy* Freya. Their respective parents occasionally offer to baby-sit, but Charlotte invariably feels too ill to go out. This is yet another bone of contention between Scott and herself.

CFS/ME sufferers with young children need a lot of practical help, and a lot of straight talking to relatives and friends is required. Charlotte cannot realistically be expected to care for a toddler all day, as well as perform other housewifely tasks – not if she wants her condition to improve. She needs to calmly inform Scott, their families and close friends of exactly how ill and miserable she feels, making it clear that, as well as daily help, she needs quality time with her child in addition to rest periods. If no one volunteers assistance (people usually do offer to help at this point) she will have no choice but to ask for it outright. She and Scott should then ask family and friends to have Freya at week-ends – maybe drawing up a rota. As the child nears nursery age, Social Services may step in to arrange early entry into nursery school.

Dorothy, John and Martin

Dorothy, 70, and John, 71, have one son, Martin, who is 44 and married with two teenage sons of his own. He is also a CFS/ME sufferer. Dorothy and John have always enjoyed holidays with Martin and his family, but they now fear that these are in jeopardy; they have proudly watched Martin's career, which he has suddenly abandoned, and they had hoped to rely on him a bit more as they grew older. They also formerly felt a sense of satisfaction at seeing him happy with his life; observing that he is now unhappy and in ill-health has even induced feelings of failure in them. Many parents measure their parenting success by the health, happiness and prosperity of their offspring.

Finding it difficult to cope with Martin's anguish, unwilling to accept that he is as incapacitated as he says he is, they constantly compare 'then' with 'now'. They see a man who has lost his 'status' in life, whose wife and sons are increasingly unhappy, and who is struggling financially because he is no longer able to provide. They make comparisons, too, with how active and alert they were at his age, how they enjoyed family life, and how they managed to care for their own ageing parents.

As Martin shows no sign of recovery, Dorothy and John's scepticism increases and they start thinking that if he 'pulls himself together' he will soon return to normal. As more time elapses, they decide that his illness is imaginary, preferring to think he is suffering from mental instability rather than from an illness they don't understand.

Martin needs to sit down with his parents and firmly assert that their attitude is hurting him. Seeing things, for the first time, from their son's viewpoint, they will probably realize that their behaviour has indeed been inappropriate. This is Martin's opportunity to tell them more about the illness, backing up his words with literature on the subject. His parents may occasionally revert to the old misconceptions, but should be willing to re-evaluate their behaviour when this is pointed out.

Self-talk

The way we speak to ourselves has great bearing on our stress levels. When we analyse our thoughts, we are often surprised at their negativity – but they must be examined before we can begin to change their destructive pattern. When the TV breaks down, for example, your initial thoughts may be, 'It's so unfair! I was really looking forward to watching that film!' 'This is all I need! I can't afford a new set!' 'Even if the set can be repaired, it will probably cost a small fortune!' 'What am I supposed to do with my time – sit twiddling my thumbs?' These are stress-provoking thoughts by any standards!

By being aware that negative thoughts create stress, you can train yourself into more positive self-talk. Using the same example, you may instead think: 'I'll ring around for quotes in the morning. Maybe it won't cost much to repair,' 'It was on its last legs anyway. I'll take the opportunity to buy a more up-to-date set,' 'I could buy a new set using hire-purchase,' 'I could buy a reconditioned set if I can't afford a new one,' 'I could rent one and not have to worry about repair costs,' 'In the meantime, this is my chance to read that book, finish my tapestry, phone Aunt Betty, etc.'

The following examples of stress-relieving self-talk can be applied to many potentially stressful situations:

'I'll break this problem into separate sections. They'll be easier to handle then.'

'Is this really worth getting upset and angry over?'

'I've coped before, so I'll cope again.'

'I can always ask for help if I need it.'

'It could have been much worse.'

'I'll take things one step at a time.'

'This is hardly a matter of life or death!'

'There's nothing I can do about this situation, so I'll have to accept it.'

5

Diet and nutrition

CFS/ME is a disorder in which the balance of the body is affected. Indeed, problems in the following systems have been found:

- *immune system* – the body's natural defence system against viral and bacterial attack;
- *central nervous system* – the many nerve tissues, located in the brain and spinal cord, that control the body's actions;
- *endocrine system* – the hormones, which are chemicals transported in bodily fluid to 'target' organs. Here they induce slow changes that lead to such things as growth, sexual development and digestion.

Because certain foods act on certain parts of the body, it has been possible to devise a diet which targets the above problem areas in CFS/ME, as discussed in this chapter.

The diet helps to support these vital systems by working from every angle possible to help the body back into balance. When the bodily systems are strengthened and once again networking properly, the errors stand a far better chance of correcting themselves.

This is far from a 'quick fix', however – it takes time for the body to heal itself. However, as long as your improved diet is a lifestyle change rather than something you do for a short time, you should soon start feeling better and have more energy.

My book *The Chronic Fatigue Healing Diet* (Sheldon Press, 2003) goes into far more detail about diet and CFS/ME. It also contains a detoxification plan, suggested daily recipe plan and a comprehensive recipe section.

Changing your food habits

Nowadays, the average Western diet is very poor. It is estimated that we eat approximately 17 per cent of our daily calories as processed foods, 18 per cent as saturated fats, 18 per cent as sugar and 3–10 per cent as alcoholic beverages. When you add this up, more than half of our foods are high in calories and low in nutrients. So it is little wonder that over time many of us develop chronic health problems.

We evolved over millions of years eating a diet that was very low in sugar and with no refined carbohydrates (such as cakes, pastries, biscuits, sweets, sweetened fruit juice, etc.). Nowadays, we tend to eat a lot of sugar, refined carbohydrates, junk foods, chemical additives and so on, and our bodies have not yet adapted – therefore our bodies treat such foods as toxic substances. Long-term use of this modern junk diet can actually result in chronic illness such as CFS/ME.

Changing the habits of a lifetime and eating a variety of food groups on a daily basis takes a lot of effort and determination. Eating is a pleasurable activity: we are used to choosing the foods that satisfy our taste buds – often made more tasty by the addition of chemical flavourings, fat, sugar, salt, etc. – and may be loathe to make drastic changes. For these reasons, I recommend that you alter your eating habits *gradually*, allowing yourself time to adjust to the new textures, appearance and flavours of different foods. With perseverance, your tastes *will* change – and as your symptoms gradually decline, your interest in the new diet will be likely to increase!

If you wish to start eating the new foods straight away, I must add a word of warning. Nutritious, cleanly grown foods may trigger the body into instant detoxification, causing headaches, lethargy and even diarrhoea, lasting between one day and two weeks. You can avoid this shock to your body by a gradual changeover.

A balanced diet such as the one outlined in this chapter can help to prevent unwanted weight gain or loss. Weight problems are common in CFS/ME because sufferers can either put on weight through inactivity or lose weight through a poor appetite related to the disorder.

A balanced wholefood diet

Wholefoods are simply those that have had nothing taken away – i.e. nutrients and fibre – and that have had nothing added – i.e. colourings, flavourings and preservatives. In short, they are foods in their most natural form. Wholefoods that are organically produced – without the use of potentially dangerous chemical fertilizers, pesticides and herbicides – are even better for us.

Fresh fruit and vegetables

People with CFS/ME often have high levels of acidity in their bodies. However, this can largely be combated by the alkalizing properties of fresh fruit and vegetables. Citrus fruits, berries, potatoes, broccoli, cauliflower, Brussels sprouts, red and green bell peppers, cabbage and spinach are also rich in vitamin C as well as other important vitamins and minerals, and this promotes a healthy immune system, among other things. Unfortunately, the vitamin C obtained from the above foods is quickly used up in the body by smoking, alcohol consumption, surgery, trauma, stress, exposure to pollutants and the use of certain medications. You should try not to eat too many tomatoes as they are highly acidic.

Fruit such as bananas, prunes, cantaloupe and honeydew melon and dried peaches and apricots are rich in potassium, which is important for good nervous system function. Potassium also helps to maintain fluid and electrolyte balance in the body.

Select locally grown organic fruit and vegetables that are in season – these have the highest nutrient content and the greatest enzyme activity. Organically grown crops may not look as perfect as those that are processed, but they *are* superior. Try to eat as fresh and as raw as possible. When you have to cook your vegetables, use unsalted (or lightly salted) water and simmer for the minimum length of time. Lightly steaming and stir-frying are healthy alternatives. Scrub rather than peel your vegetables.

Some other eating suggestions are listed below:

- Eat a range of different fruits to add more interest. Different fruits provide different nutrients.
- If you work, pack an orange, banana or grapes to snack on during the day.
- Dried apricots, peaches and pineapple slices store well, so you can keep a bag of them in your drawer at work to snack on.
- Add crushed fresh pineapple to coleslaw and cottage cheese and add mandarin oranges or grapes to a tossed salad.
- Have baked apples, pears or a fruit salad for dessert.
- When buying tinned fruit, choose fruit soaked in 100 per cent fruit juice rather than syrup.
- Make a variety of green salads and try to eat one every day.
- Vary your vegetables to make your meals more interesting.
- Buy packets of baby carrots or celery sticks to snack on.
- To make a quick meal when you aren't feeling too good, it's okay to buy tinned vegetables. Look for labels saying 'no salt added'. If you feel you then need to add a small pinch of salt yourself, it will still amount to far less than that in a normal tin of vegetables.
- Plan some meals around vegetables rather than around meat. Examples are vegetable stir-fry, vegetable curry and vegetable soup.

- Add chopped vegetables to a pasta sauce or lasagne.
- To thicken and flavour a soup, stew or gravy, use cooked and pureed vegetables such as potatoes.
- When preparing a barbecue meal, try grilled vegetable kebabs.

Legumes (peas and beans)

Legumes are very cheap to buy and contain high amounts of protein, which is vital to the body for growth and maintenance. Protein is directly responsible for approximately 20 per cent of the material in our tissues and cells, and it functions as hormones, antibodies and enzymes, all of which keep the body functioning smoothly. Protein also helps to relieve stiffness and pain.

The soya bean is a complete protein, of which there are many derivatives including soya milk, tofu, tempeh and miso. Tofu, for example, is very versatile and can be used in both savoury and sweet dishes. Soya milk can be used as an alternative to cow's milk.

Seeds

Sunflower, sesame, hemp, flax and pumpkin seeds are very important for strengthening the immune system. They can be eaten as they are as a snack, sprinkled onto salads and cereals, or used in baking. For more flavour they can be lightly roasted and coated with organic soy sauce. Cracked linseed and pumpkin seeds are also highly nutritious and useful for treating constipation. They can be used in baking and sprinkled onto breakfast cereals or over salads, soups and porridge oats.

Nuts

Nuts, too, are an intrinsic part of strengthening the immune system. All nuts contain vital nutrients, but almonds, cashews, walnuts, Brazils and pecans perhaps offer the greatest array. Eat a wide assortment as snacks, with cereal and in baking. Obviously, if you are allergic to nuts, they must be avoided at all costs.

Grains

Wholegrain and wholemeal flours provide us with the complex unrefined carbohydrates our bodies require – and again organic is best. Many types of grain are good for us, but wheat – our staple in the West – contains gluten and can be highly allergenic for some people. You can find out whether you are allergic or sensitive to wheat by following the food elimination diet as described on pages 75–6. Although nutritious, wheat is also an acidic food, which is not recommended for people with CFS/ME as the body is likely to be over-acidic already, as mentioned earlier.

With the exception of wheat, aim to consume a variety of grains, including oats, rye, barley (generally available as pearl barley), corn, buckwheat, brown rice and mixed grains. Brown rice, millet, buckwheat and maize/corn are all gluten-free and invaluable to people with a gluten allergy or sensitivity.

Oats are particularly beneficial as not only do they provide a slow release of energy, which helps to stabilize blood sugar levels, they also nourish the central nervous system and are rich in minerals and the B vitamins. Therefore they help the body to normalize itself and reduce its over-reaction to the normal environmental substances to which many people with CFS/ME are sensitive.

Here are some further tips for eating wholegrain:

- Try to eat a bowl of porridge for breakfast every day; buy oatmeal biscuits and oat cereal bars.
- Use brown rice instead of white.
- If you can eat wheat, use wholewheat pasta instead of refined white pasta.
- Use wholegrains such as barley in soups and stews.
- Use bulgur wheat in casseroles and stir-fries.
- Make a pilaf with wholegrains such as wild rice, brown rice and barley.
- Substitute half the refined white flour in pancakes, buns and other flour-based recipes for wholewheat or oat flour.
- Use rolled oats or crushed unsweetened wholegrain cereal to bread chicken, fish, veal cutlets, and so on.
- Use wholegrain flour or oatmeal when making baked treats.
- As the colour of a grain is not an indication of whether it is 'whole' or not, read the ingredient list.

Fats and oils

Fats (fatty acids) are the most concentrated sources of energy in our diet, one gram of fat providing the body with nine calories of energy. They are also a fine source of essential fatty acids (EFAs) which improve circulation and oxygen uptake. Our bodies are unable to manufacture EFAs, so they can only come from our diets. A deficiency in EFAs is linked with muscle tissue-wasting, reduced immune-system function and diminished cognitive ability.

There are two distinct types of fatty acids – one bad, one good:

- *Saturated fat* – Believed to be implicated in the development of heart disease, saturated fat comes mainly from animal sources and is generally solid at room temperature. Although margarine was for many years believed to be a healthier choice over butter, nutritionists have now revised their opinion, for some of the fats in the margarine hydrogenation process are changed into trans-fatty acids which the body metabolizes as if they were saturated fatty acids – the same as butter. Butter is a valuable source of oils and vitamin A, but should be used very sparingly. Margarine, on the other hand, is an artificial product containing many additives, which are not recommended in CFS/ME.
- *Unsaturated fat* – Also called polyunsaturated or monounsaturated fat, unsaturated fat has a protective effect on the heart and other organs. Omega 3 and omega 6 oils occur naturally in oily fish (mackerel, herring, sardines, tuna, etc.), nuts and seeds, and is usually liquid at room temperature. It is recommended, then, that people with CFS/ME eat oily fish at least three times a week and cold-pressed oil (olive, rapeseed, safflower and sunflower oil) daily, for dressings and in cooking.

Cow's milk products

Cow's milk products include cheese, yogurt, cream, butter, ice-cream, condensed milk, evaporated milk and powdered milk – all of which are rich in calcium, protein and the vitamins A, D and E. However, little trace of these vitamins remains after the pasteurization process and they are often replaced (fortified) by dairies in harmful amounts. Moreover, the protein in cow's milk products is comprised of 80 per cent casein and 20 per cent whey, which both have allergenic properties. Cow's milk products also contain a lot of the sugar lactose – indeed, a glass of milk contains as much as half the sugar in a glass of a fizzy drink. Unfortunately, lactose is difficult for many people to digest and can cause sensitivity problems. In fact, it is believed that up to 75 per cent of the world's population suffer from a degree of lactose intolerance, the symptoms of which include bloating, stomach aches and diarrhoea. People with CFS/ME seem to be particularly vulnerable.

The calcium in cow's milk products is the best thing about it. What you may not know is that sufficient calcium can be obtained from regular consumption of dark leafy vegetables, seaweed (kelp, wakame and hijiki), nuts and seeds, beans, oranges and figs. As calcium is essential to the development of strong bones and teeth in children – who are less likely to enjoy eating the above calcium alternatives on a regular basis – cow's milk should only be removed from their diet if they have allergy problems or lactose intolerance.

Below is some further advice related to cow's milk products:

- Full-fat 'whole milk' products contain a good deal of saturated fat, which can be harmful to our arteries, especially in large amounts. If you must drink milk, choose fat-free (skimmed) or low-fat. Cow's milk produce should also be low-fat.

- If possible, buy 'tuberculin-tested' milk instead of pasteurized, particularly if you don't have lactose intolerance or an allergy to the casein and whey in milk.

- Cow's milk often contains bovine growth hormone, antibiotics and pesticides, which may be responsible for some of the health problems linked to milk.

- If you have lactose intolerance but enjoy milk products, choose lactose-free alternatives. There is lactose-free yogurt and cheese, as well as lactose-free milk. Alternatively, you could try taking the enzyme lactase before consuming milk products to reduce or eliminate intolerance symptoms. Ask at your local health shop about this.

- To eliminate the risk attached to cow's milk and other dairy produce, you can cut it out altogether. With the exception of vitamin D, all the vitamins and minerals obtained from cow's milk products are found in foods that are part of a healthy balanced diet. Vitamin D is obtained from sunlight – however, if you don't seem to get a lot of that and would like to stop consuming cow's milk products, take a vitamin D supplement.

- Alternatives to cow's milk include (calcium-enriched) soya milk, rice milk, coconut milk, almond milk, goat's milk and sheep milk (goat and sheep milk are a lot less allergenic than cow's milk).

- If you are eliminating milk products from your diet, ensure that you replace them with oil-containing foods such as oily fish, nuts and seeds.

- Beans, pulses, soya, fish and poultry products can give us all the protein our bodies require. Sufficient protein is essential in CFS/ME as it helps to relieve stiffness and pain.

- If you don't consume milk products, you can ensure you have enough calcium by buying calcium fortified cereals, breads, soy drinks, rice drinks and fruit juices.

Eggs

Contrary to popular belief, the cholesterol in eggs is not now thought to be a risk factor in arterial disease. Indeed, research has shown that egg cholesterol has a clinically insignificant effect on levels of blood cholesterol. Eggs also contain lecithin, a superb biological detergent capable of breaking down fats so they can be utilized by the body. In addition, lecithin prevents the accumulation of too many acid or alkaline substances in the blood and encourages the transport of nutrients through the cell walls. Buy free-range eggs and eat them soft-boiled or poached, as a hard yolk will bind the lecithin, rendering it useless as a fat-detergent.

The Food Standards Agency now states that most people don't need to limit their consumption of eggs so long as they are part of a balanced diet.

Red meat

As red meat is often loaded with saturated fat, it should be eaten in moderation. Look for organically produced meat as the use of pesticides, antibiotics and hormones in animal husbandry is an ongoing health issue. If you can't bear to go without red meat, make your serving no larger or thicker than the palm of your hand, and don't eat red meat more than three times a week.

Unfortunately, reducing your consumption of red meat will lower your protein intake (which needs to be fairly high in a CFS/ME diet). You should therefore ensure that you eat sufficient alternative protein-containing foods such as fish, poultry, soya products, cottage cheese, organic live yogurt, nuts, seeds and legumes. Also, if you eat a lot of grain products such as bread, pasta, rice and cereals, you are unlikely to be consuming enough protein and this can lead to further weakening of the immune system. Low protein intake causes the body to pull protein from the muscles, and this causes further weakness, low energy, low stamina, poor resistance to infection and depression. Protein deficiency symptoms are strongly linked with CFS/ME.

Here are some suggestions for buying, cooking and eating red meat:

- Choose the leanest cuts of meat you can find. The leanest beef cuts include top loin, top sirloin and shoulder. The leanest pork cuts include pork loin, tenderloin and ham. The leanest lamb cuts are from the shank half of the leg.
- Trim away the visible fat before cooking.
- Grill, roast, poach or boil red meat instead of frying.

- If you must fry your meat on the odd occasion, don't bread it as the bread adds fat and causes the meat to soak up even more fat.
- Choose extra lean minced meat.
- Any fat that arises from cooking should be carefully drained off.
- Hams, sausages, frankfurters, burgers and luncheon meats are processed and contain added sodium (salt). Unless it says 'low sodium content' on the label, they should be avoided.
- As lower-fat processed meats are now in the shops, check out the nutrition facts on the label and choose those with less fat and saturated fat.

Fish

Fish is a nutritious alternative to red meat. It is particularly beneficial as it is an excellent source of omega 3 fatty acids and gamma linoleic acid (GLA), deficiencies of which can encourage inflammation and so aggravate feverishness, aches and pains. Fish is also a great source of the amino acids your body needs to build protein. Choose cold-water fish, especially oily fish such as sardines, fresh tuna, anchovies, mackerel, trout, salmon, herring (kippers) and pilchards.

- Avoid frying fish. Poach, grill or bake instead.
- Avoid covering fish in breadcrumbs, as this adds more fat and makes the fish soak up additional fat.

Poultry

Poultry such as chicken and turkey contains far less fat than red meat and is a good source of protein and essential fatty acids (EFAs). EFAs can improve circulation and oxygen uptake. It is therefore recommended that you eat chicken or turkey once or twice a week.

- The leanest poultry choices are boneless chicken breasts and turkey cutlets.
- Fresh chicken and turkey is usually 'flavour-enhanced' by the use of sodium (salt). Avoid poultry with 'self-basting' on the label as this is an indication of sodium addition.
- Even better, look for 'organic' and 'free range' on the label.

Sprouted foods

When foods are sprouted, dormant enzymes spring into action, providing more nutrients per gram than any other natural food. They can therefore be a great help in normalizing all the body's systems. Eating a mixture of different sprouts is even capable of supporting life on its own – although this is not recommended! You may wish to try sprouting seeds and beans and eating them yourself.

Fresh seeds, beans and grains will sprout when rinsed and placed in pure water in a plastic bowl or polythene bag. The container should be sealed and placed in an airing cupboard or by a radiator for three or four days, the liquid being changed twice a day. A dose of light and sunshine will make them ready for eating. *Be very aware, though, that seed potatoes and tomatoes should not be sprouted – they belong to the deadly nightshade family. Kidney bean sprouts are poisonous, too.*

Eat your sprouted foods in salads and soups.

Foods to avoid

It is known that reducing or eliminating the foods mentioned in this section can improve CFS/ME symptoms.

Salt

Because of its ability to inhibit the growth of harmful micro-organisms, high levels of salt are added as a preservative to most processed and pre-packaged foods. For example, one tin of soup contains more salt (sodium) than the recommended daily allowance for an adult. Large amounts of salt are also added to most breakfast cereals, except for Shredded Wheat products.

It is recommended, therefore, that you limit your intake of salt in the following ways:

- Reduce your consumption of processed and pre-packaged foods, as mentioned earlier.
- When you must buy processed and pre-packaged foods, look for 'low-salt' or 'sodium-free' on the label.
- Use only a very small amount of sea salt or rock salt in baking and cooking.
- Try to avoid sprinkling any type of salt over your meals.

Reducing your salt intake very gradually is the best way to retrain your palate.

Sugar

Sugar consumption has been linked with many disorders, from diabetes to heart disease and cancer. We do need a certain amount of sugar in our diets for conversion to energy, but that can be obtained naturally from foods such as fruits and complex carbohydrates.

If you really must sweeten your food and drinks, alternatives to refined white sugar include raw honey and barley malt. Muscovado and demerara (both of which may be referred to as 'soft brown sugar') are formed during the early stages of the sugar refining process and so contain more nutrients than refined white sugar. The above-mentioned can all be used in cooking and baking.

Please note that it is not advisable to replace refined white sugar with a sugar substitute such as aspartame, which is sold under the brand names of NutraSweet, Spoonful, Equal and Indulge. Aspartame is an excitatory neuro (nerve)-transmitter that causes nerve cells to fire continually until they become exhausted and die – and of course this is not at all good for general health. Unfortunately, many people consume food and drinks containing aspartame in an attempt to lose weight. You may be surprised to learn, though, that this artificial sweetener creates a craving for simple carbohydrates such as cakes, pastries, biscuits and so on, which only gives rise to an increase in weight. When the person stops using aspartame – in diet drinks, for example – he or she generally loses weight. Fortunately, there are natural sweeteners such as Stevia and Xylitol that are perfectly safe and available from health food shops.

Caffeine

Caffeine products – which include coffee, tea, cocoa, cola drinks, energy drinks and chocolate – cause adrenal gland exhaustion, which makes it difficult for the body to cope with stress. The adrenal glands are tired and weakened anyway in CFS/ME, and continuing to use stimulants of any kind only makes the situation worse. Caffeine products are also toxic to the liver, are detrimental to the nervous system and can reduce the body's ability to absorb vitamins and minerals. Consumed regularly in fairly high doses, they are likely to give rise to chronic anxiety, the symptoms of which are agitation, palpitations, headaches, indigestion, panic, insomnia and hyperventilation. My best advice is to remove caffeine products from your diet.

The addictiveness of caffeine makes reduction far from easy, however, and withdrawal symptoms can take the form of splitting headaches, fatigue, depression, poor concentration and muscle pains. It's no wonder people can feel terrible until they have had their first dose of caffeine in the morning, and that they can't seem to function properly without regular doses throughout the day! Fortunately, caffeine is quickly 'washed out' of the system – and it is possible to minimize withdrawal symptoms by reducing intake over several weeks.

A problem for many is finding an acceptable alternative. Coffee, tea, cocoa and cola drinks can be replaced by fruit juices, vegetable juices and herbal teas. Of these, green tea is very good, as is rooibosch (redbush) tea; both are low in tannin and high in beneficial antioxidants. A variety of grain coffee substitutes may also be purchased from health food shops. Because many decaffeinated products are processed with the use of chemicals, they are, unfortunately, not a good choice.

Carob, which is similar to the cocoa bean, is a healthy, caffeine-free alternative to cocoa and chocolate. It contains less fat and is naturally sweet, unlike the cocoa bean which is bitter and needs sweetening. Many people find carob bars an enjoyable replacement for chocolate bars and other confectionery. Carob is also available in powder form for use in baking and in drinks.

Artificial colourings

Many of today's processed foods contain artificial colourings such as tartrazine to make them more appealing to the customer. However, food colourings are derived from petroleum and contain toxic compounds that have been linked to many diseases. If you really must buy processed foods, remember to read the list of ingredients to ensure that there are no artificial colourings. It's always best to buy fresh foods.

Other stimulants to avoid

Two of the main reasons that human beings crave stimulants such as caffeine (see page 72), cigarettes, alcohol and products containing refined white sugar (see page 71) are feelings of exhaustion and high levels of stress. When CFS/ME symptoms make you feel worn out and stressed, your body demands a boost of energy – a 'lift'. However, the lift obtained from stimulants is short-lived, unlike the damage it can do to your adrenal glands, which are already tired and weakened in CFS/ME. Stimulants can also create a hypersensitive immune system, chronic anxiety, low energy, nerve cell damage and many more things, most of which are already part and parcel of CFS/ME and are commonly made worse by stimulant use.

If you find you are unable to completely eliminate stimulants from your diet, reduce them as much as possible – it *will* make a difference.

Alcohol

Many CFS/ME sufferers cannot tolerate alcohol, some saying it causes their blood to feel like acid in their veins. Also, it appears that the more some sufferers drink, the more severe their symptoms become. These responses point to poor liver function, which can actually be tested for; please ask your doctor about this.

Unfortunately, alcohol – a toxin – acts on the central nervous system, which is often highly sensitized in CFS/ME anyway. As herbal tinctures usually contain small amounts of alcohol, they too may not be tolerated by individuals who are especially sensitive.

Because antioxidants are required to mop up the damaging free radicals stimulated by the liver's alcohol detoxification process, alcohol consumption can deplete antioxidant supplies. Even more damaging is the fact that pesticides, colourants and other harmful additives are generally involved in modern-day alcohol production, exerting further strain on the liver. For these reasons, even people who do not have an immediate adverse reaction to alcohol would be best advised to avoid it.

Smoking

If you smoke, you don't need me or anyone else to tell you it's not good for you. What you may not know is that smoking is particularly harmful in CFS/ME. This is because a condition known as Multiple Chemical Sensitivities (MCS) is closely linked to CFS/ME, and commercial cigarettes are loaded with chemicals. The main ones are benzene, formaldehyde, ammonia and acetone – but actually a massive 600 toxic chemicals are absorbed into your bloodstream with every single inhalation.

Chemicals are often responsible for a flare-up of CFS/ME; they can also cause the nerve-ending inflammation present in CFS/ME. There's no hope of recovery or even symptom stability if you continue to introduce toxic chemicals into your body.

Some people with CFS/ME say that smoking helps to deal with the stress of the condition and generally lowers their pain levels. Of course, this is difficult to get past in an emotional sense. However, when weighed against the damage the chemicals in cigarettes do to your body, the trade-off has a very high price. Indeed, it is virtually impossible to recover from CFS/ME without stopping smoking.

The food elimination diet

Although most adverse reactions to foods are a result of food 'intolerance', we tend to think of all food reactions as 'allergies'. The main difference between intolerance and allergy is that an intolerance reaction can take up to 24 hours to present itself, whereas a true allergy provokes an immediate reaction and can vary from a headache to anaphylactic shock, which is a life-threatening condition.

Food elimination

You may already have a fairly good idea of which foods your body cannot tolerate. If not, keep a careful record of the foods you eat and note any reactions. When you have a clearer idea of the culprits, eliminate them from your diet for a period of one month. Ensure that you replace any dairy products you eliminate with sufficient protein, and oil-containing foods and wheat products with alternative grains.

If you suspect you are sensitive to several different foods, it's advisable that you attend an 'allergy'-testing clinic. There are many 'allergy'-friendly foods and supplements available from health food shops, as well as from certain pharmacies.

When the offending foods are first withdrawn, there is occasionally an initial withdrawal reaction, producing such symptoms as fatigue, headaches, twitching and irritability for up to 15 days. Drinking as much water as possible will help to reduce these symptoms. It also aids detoxification, helping to flush any residual offending foods through the system.

Reintroduction strategy

Towards the end of the month you may feel better than you have for a long time! The feeling of well-being can be so great you won't want to bother reintroducing the excluded foods.

However, for those who do wish to reintroduce those foods, the following procedure is suggested:

Day 1   In the morning, reintroduce a small amount of *one* of the foods eliminated (not a full-sized portion). Do the same later in the day. Record any symptoms.

Day 2   If you experienced no symptoms, repeat the exercise. Once again, record any symptoms. If you get through the second day, this is really good news! Now wait for two days before you can safely reintroduce this food into your diet on a fairly regular basis.

Repeat the above four-day reintroduction procedure with each food eliminated. Any side-effects should have occurred within four days. If you do experience symptoms – say, for example, you develop a headache after reintroducing tomatoes – it would be better to leave tomatoes alone for at least six months before making another attempt to reintroduce them. However, some foods may always cause an adverse reaction and it would be wise to withdraw them from your diet altogether.

You may be disappointed, too, if your problem is true allergy. In such instances, the offending food provokes an immediate reaction, i.e. the immune system responds as if it is being invaded, setting up anti-bodies to the food in question. Obviously you will need to continue avoiding this food. Dairy products are the top food allergen and wheat the second. If you find you are sensitive to either of these (or both) make sure you replace them with plenty of protein and oil-containing foods and/or alternative grains.

Nutritional supplements

World-famous immunologist Dr Robert Good stated that a moderate and steady calorie intake combined with the right nutrients fortifies the immune system and aids in fighting disease. As people with CFS/ME have suppressed immune systems, it is important that they boost the benefits of a balanced diet (as described earlier in this chapter) with vitamin and mineral supplements.

Vitamin and mineral supplements

- *Vitamin C (ascorbic acid)* – In a depressed immune system there is a shortfall of ascorbic acid, which is an excellent detoxifier and helps to reduce stress. Take up to 3000 mg of vitamin C daily.
- *Vitamin B complex* – As the B group of vitamins helps to reduce anxiety and stress, it is best to take a high-potency B-complex supplement twice daily.
- *Vitamin E* – As vitamin E helps to improve sleep, alleviate fatigue, boost healing and aid in the utilization of vitamin A by the body, you can take up to 400 IU daily.
- *Vitamin A (beta-carotene, the precursor to retinol)* – This vitamin is necessary for the growth and repair of all the bodily tissues. Take up to 10,000 IU per day.
- *NADH (nicotinamide adenine dinucleotide)* – Derived from vitamin B3, this coenzyme enables the body to increase adenine triphosphate (ATP), the fuel that provides the body with energy. NADH also helps

to boost the immune system. Take 15–30 mg daily, depending upon the severity of symptoms. The dosage should be reduced to 5 mg per day when symptoms improve.

- *Calcium* – This is the most abundant mineral in the body, 99 per cent of it being found in the bones and teeth. It works with magnesium to ensure proper muscle contraction/relaxations, and is important to nervous system function. Take up to 1000 mg daily.
- *Magnesium* – This mineral is important for the absorption of calcium, phosphorous, potassium, vitamins C and E, and the B-complex vitamins, and it aids the conversion of blood sugar to energy. Take 600–1200 mg daily.
- *Manganese* – This mineral helps to create energy from glucose. It also aids in the normalization of the central nervous system. Take up to 10 mg daily.
- *Zinc* – This mineral is involved in a wide range of metabolic activities, including digestion, protein synthesis and insulin production. It is also required for good immune system function. Take up to 15 mg daily.
- *Selenium* – This mineral protects helps to boost the immune system. Take up to 100 mcg daily.
- *Potassium* – Together with sodium, this mineral works to regulate heart and muscle function. It also ensures the correct acid/alkaline balance; normal transmission of nerve impulses; stability of internal cell structure and stimulation of the kidneys to eliminate toxic body waste. Take up to 5000 mg daily.
- *Chromium* – This mineral works with the B vitamins and magnesium to metabolize sugar and stabilize blood sugar levels. As chromium is lost in the urine whenever sugar is consumed, a high sugar intake can lead to chromium deficiency. Take up to 67 mg daily.

Other useful supplements

- *Malic acid* – This supplement plays a vital role in the operation of the 'malic acid shuttle service', which delivers important nutrients to the cells for conversion to energy. It is particularly effective when combined with magnesium. Some supplement manufacturers now offer magnesium malate, which combines the two. Take up to 200 mg daily.
- *Co-enzyme Q10* – This enzyme is an important aid to people with CFS/ME as it helps to increase mental and physical energy and alleviate fatigue. It works by aiding the transfer of oxygen and energy between components of the cells and between the blood and the tissues. Take up to 100 mg daily.

- *Boron* – This trace element is thought to be involved in bone min-eralization, and is important to maintaining good muscular health. Because people with CFS/ME may be inactive for long periods, it can also reduce calcium loss. Take up to 3 mg daily.

Guidance on taking supplements

As vitamins A, C and E (known as the 'ACE' vitamins) together with CoQ10, selenium, zinc and manganese work as fine antioxidants (a compound that removes potentially damaging agents from the body), they should be your first line of defence. These substances can be purchased together in a single high-potency antioxidant supplement from specialist suppliers and sold under brand names such as Revenol, NutriGuard Plus or Resveratrol. The constituents may be also bought separately, but at a higher overall price. Trials have shown that the above-mentioned combination of antioxidants should be taken for a period of one month before commencing further supplementation. However, B-complex supplementation and Evening Primrose Oil could be started after two weeks.

During Month 2 I suggest that you begin taking one of the adap-togenic herbs. For instance, *rhodiola rosea*, Siberian ginseng and ashwagandha help to normalize and regulate the various systems within the body, promoting health and well-being. You could then start magnesium and malic acid supplementation. These substances work together to reduce fatigue, pain and low muscle stamina. In the main, they can only be bought separately but, as mentioned earlier, certain specialist suppliers sell magnesium malate, a compound of the two.

A multi-mineral and trace element supplement containing calcium, magnesium, manganese, zinc, potassium and chromium should also be taken after a further two weeks. Most people find that a liquid for-mulation gives greater absorption than the tablet form – e.g. Maximol. (See the Useful Addresses section for information about a supplier of nutritional supplements.)

During Month 3, you may wish to begin taking *ginkgo biloba* and CoQ10, which work to improve brain function and energy production. However, check that these nutrients are not already included in your antioxidant preparation. Echinacea, the immune system stimulant, could be sampled for reaction in Month 4 – most people are able to tolerate it.

Unfortunately, because of the many deficiencies in CFS/ME, sup-plementation is important. By following the diet alone, you should, in time, see a noticeable difference in your health – but by incorporating the recommended supplements you give your body an even greater chance of healing. Having said that, please remember that to take only one or two supplements is better than none at all. The antioxidant preparation is of prime importance, as is magnesium malate, closely followed by the liquid mineral and trace element formulation.

It is important to note that when you start taking a course of supplements, your body may begin to detoxify straight away, releasing stored toxins and debris into the bloodstream. This may cause headaches and lethargy for a day or so, until the loosened toxins are eliminated from the body. Try not to be overly concerned about this, for it's a sure sign that you are on your way to better health.

Chemical sensitivities

People with CFS/ME are particularly susceptible to chemical stressors which enter the body through the skin, nasal passages and digestive tract. The constant onslaught of chemicals greatly stresses the detoxification organs, causing sluggish liver function and immune system impairment. As a result, infections can linger and fatigue may persist. In time, the immune system may even begin to react against the chemicals themselves, perhaps causing hives, itching, skin eruptions, runny nose, sneezing, diarrhoea, tinnitus, cramps, excessive fatigue, respiratory problems and confusion.

Indoor air contaminants include building materials, paints, varnish, glues, deodorants, plastics, carpeting, insecticides, disinfectants, detergents, dyes and gas leakage from stoves and heaters. Personal care products such as deodorants, skin lotions, cosmetics, perfumes, shower gels, hair shampoo and conditioners can also provoke adverse reactions in sensitive individuals. Biologically friendly products are now available from certain high-street chemists, and from some suppliers of nutritional supplements.

Outdoor contaminants include industrial fumes, traffic exhaust fumes, smog, crop-spraying and the paving and resurfacing of roads. Synthetic drugs – that is, those derived from petroleum – are also a common source of sensitivity. The colourings and flavourings in medications and foods can cause problems, too.

Avoiding exposure to the chemicals which cause you a problem will doubtlessly improve your condition. Following the diet recommended in this chapter, as well as use of the recommended nutritional supplements, is also important, and can reduce chemical sensitivity.

The most common chemical sensitivities include the following:

- *Organophosphates* – These chemicals are widely used in farming practices for pest control and animal husbandry, causing many of the symptoms linked with CFS/ME. They are also used in home pesticides such as fly sprays, etc. You can detox your body of organophosphates by following an organic diet, and by taking antioxidant supplements. Vitamins A, C and E, vitamin B12, magnesium and selenium are particularly effective.
- *Aluminium* – Because high levels of aluminium damage the central nervous system, this chemical is believed to be highly implicated in the evolution and persistence of CFS/ME. Avoid using aluminium containers, foil wrap and underarm deodorants which contain aluminium salts.
- *Mercury* – People with amalgam tooth fillings are ingesting minute amounts of mercury vapour every day. This can gradually weaken the immune system in sensitive individuals. Some think ingested mercury vapour may even cause CFS/ME – it certainly causes similar symptoms. Synthetic white fillings are a safe alternative.
- *Lead* – Ingested lead is known to cause neurological and psychological disturbance. Some old houses still have lead piping while others have copper piping fused together with lead-based solder. The use of a water-filter is highly recommended in cases like this although, obviously, replacing the old piping with modern copper or synthetic piping is far safer.
- *Cadmium* – High carbohydrate consumption is now thought to be linked with high cadmium levels in the body. Cigarette-smoking is another cause of cadmium build-up, cadmium being mainly absorbed through the lungs. This metal is known to be damaging to the kidneys and lungs. It can, however, be gradually removed by good nutrition and giving up the 'weed', if you smoke.

Water

Experts believe the thirst reflex is often suppressed in people with CFS/ME, causing too little intake of fluids. In addition, research has shown that the red blood cells of sufferers become sticky and clump together, which emphasizes the need for adequate water consumption. However, whether tap water is suitable for human consumption is a matter for debate. Water in the UK is thought to be superior to that in a number of other countries, but it is still laden with toxic chemicals and inorganic salts which are undoubtedly detrimental to people with CFS/ME.

In areas of 'hard' water, where rainwater has run through limestone (containing sodium salts and calcium salts) our tap water has a high mineral content, particularly of mineral salts. This can cause fluid retention and a concentration of salts in our tissues. Ultimately, it can even lead to high blood pressure and hardening of the arteries. 'Soft' water, on the other hand, is usually filtered through sandstone and peat, which removes many of the impurities. This is better, until chemicals are added, such as chlorine and, in some areas, fluoride.

As you can see, our tap water can end up being saturated with inappropriate mineral salts and added chemicals. If you are interested in the water consistency in your postal area, the Water Authority will provide a breakdown upon request. As tap water is certainly of some detriment to people with CFS/ME, I recommend that you use a good water filter or buy bottled uncarbonated spring water.

6

Exercise

Perhaps the most important treatment for CFS/ME is exercise – and yet exercise is often the most difficult thing for sufferers to do. The condition usually means that you find yourself in a vicious downward spiral of increasing fatigue and increasing amounts of rest. The prolonged periods of rest your body demands inevitably lead to muscle wasting, which in turn leads to decreased performance. As a result, it is common to become disillusioned about life in general and thus to have no interest in even trying to exercise.

However, taking a small amount of exercise every day and very gradually increasing your levels of activity can put a halt to the downward spiral and slowly but surely replace it with a new and far more positive upward spiral. This leads to improved muscle tone, more energy, feelings of optimism and therefore greater interest in exercise. In other words, the more exercise you do, the better you feel and the more you want to do.

I can't emphasize enough the positive psychological effects of regular exercise. Indeed, it has been shown in studies to reduce anxiety, improve well-being and act as an antidepressant. This is because carrying out any kind of exercise produces natural feel-good chemicals called endorphins which give you a 'lift'. Regular exercise also helps to keep your bones strong, it maintains joint mobility and is of great benefit to the lungs and cardiovascular system.

Carrying out a daily exercise routine can also help in the following ways:

- It will reduce your levels of stress – and stress is one of the exacerbating factors in CFS/ME.
- It stimulates the lymph glands, which operate as a sewage system to rid the body of harmful toxins. The flow of lymph from the lymph glands is entirely dependent upon muscular movement.
- It can increase the body's tolerance of chemicals in the environment.
- It can help you to sleep better at night, which in turn means that you wake feeling more refreshed the next morning.
- It gives a real sense of achievement – not least because you are undoing the damage to your muscles and increasing their endurance and strength.

How to get started

Many people with CFS/ME have had bad experiences of trying some form of exercise, which has put them off trying again. The key is to start with extreme care and to only pick the exercises you think you can comfortably do. When first attempting to exercise, you may experience a faster heart-beat, faster breathing and perhaps some muscle tension afterwards. These are normal reactions in an unfit person and mean that your body is making the necessary adjustments. Muscles that have wasted are bound to be tight, and the only way to stretch and strengthen them is to exercise. Without exercise your body is liable to become increasingly fatigued and painful.

If you have joint and/or muscle pain that lasts for more than three hours after exercising, or if your pain and fatigue are worse the next day, you know you have done too much. Wait a few days for your body to recover, then make the following changes:

- Choose less demanding exercises for your routine.
- Reduce the number of repetitions.
- Perform your routine more gently and at a slower pace.

Because the severity of CFS/ME symptoms varies considerably from person to person, it is best for each individual to develop a personalized routine. This routine should depend largely upon which activities you are most able to do without provoking additional fatigue and pain.

As you read through the exercise possibilities, make a list of the ones you think you may be able to do. Although only 'warm-ups' may be within your scope at the outset, you may be able to expand your routine as your muscles gain in flexibility and strength.

Warm-up exercises

Some of your muscles may be permanently tight and prone to being painful. If you try to move them beyond a certain point, they may resist, and forcing them only makes them more painful. It is essential, therefore, that before attempting to strengthen such muscles, you perform warm-up exercises at the start of your routine. Warm-ups should include mobility exercises for your joints, simple pulse-raising activities for your heart and lungs, and short static stretches for your muscles. One or two repetitions of several exercises are generally better than several repetitions of only one or two exercises. Never skip warm-ups in favour of more vigorous exercise.

Mobility exercises

These exercises should be smooth and continuous. It is important, too, that you keep your body relaxed. Exercising when tense can cause more harm than good. Remember to keep your back straight, your bottom tucked in and your stomach flattened as you perform your routine. You should stand with your legs slightly apart.

Shoulders   Letting your arms hang loose, slowly circle your shoulders backwards. Repeat the exercise between two and ten times, depending upon the severity of your condition. Now slowly circle your shoulders forwards and repeat between two and ten times.

Neck (1)   Making sure you are standing straight, slowly turn your head to the left as far as it will comfortably go, then hold to a count of two. Return to centre and repeat the exercise between two and ten times. Now turn your head to the right, holding to a count of two before returning to centre. Repeat between two and ten times.

Neck (2)   Tucking in your chin a little, tilt your head down and hold to a count of two. Repeat between two and ten times. Again tucking in your chin a little, lift your head upward – but not so far that it virtually sits on your shoulders – and hold to a count of two. Repeat between two and ten times.

Spine (1)   Placing your hands on your hips to help support your lower back, slowly tilt your upper body to the left and hold to a count of two. Return to centre, and repeat between two and ten times. Now tilt to the right and return to centre. Repeat between two and ten times (see Figure 1).

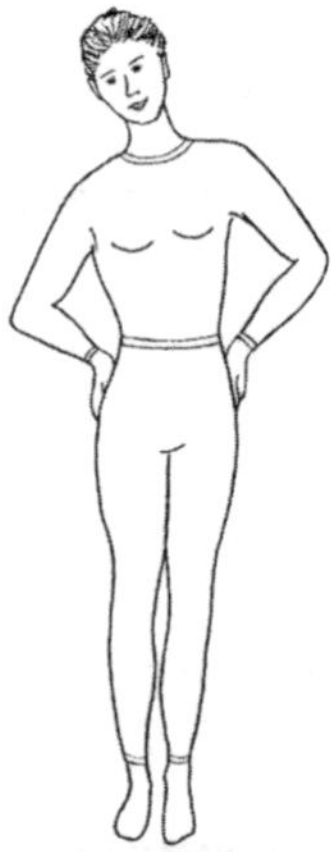

Spine (2)   Keeping your lower back static, swing your arms and upper body to the left as far as it will comfortably go, then return to centre. Repeat between two and ten times. Now swing your arms and upper body to the right and return to centre. Repeat between two and ten times

Hips and knees   With your body upright, move your hips by lifting your left knee upward, as far

Figure 1

as is comfortable. Hold to a count of two, then lower. Now raise your right knee and hold to a count of two. Repeat between two and ten times (see Figure 2).

Ankles   With your right leg slightly bent, place your left heel on the floor in front of you. Lift up your foot and then place your left toes on the floor. Repeat between two and ten times. Now duplicate the exercise and number of repetitions with the right foot (see Figures 3a and 3b).

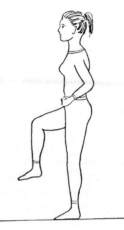

Figure 2

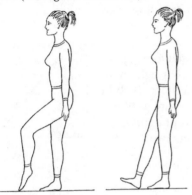

Figures 3(a) and (b)

Pulse-raising activities

Still part of your warm-up routine, pulse-raising activities must be gentle and should build up very gradually. Their purpose is to help warm your muscles in preparation for stretching. Walking around the room for two to four minutes followed, if possible, by walking once up and down the stairs, is ideal.

Stretching exercises

Muscles that are already becoming warm and flexible relax further when you perform short stretches followed by mobility and pulse-raising activities. The following stretching exercises have been devised with the help of the Health Education Authority.

Again, it is up to you to decide which you think you are capable of performing. On days when you feel more delicate than usual, carrying out a few stretching exercises rather than performing your entire routine should help to relax the muscles.

Calf (1) Stand with your arms outstretched in front of you and your palms against a wall. Keeping your left foot on the floor, bend your left knee. Press the heel of your right foot into the floor until you feel a gentle stretch in your leg muscles. Now alternate legs and repeat between two and ten times (see Figure 4).

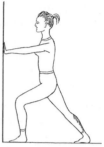

Calf (2) Standing with your feet slightly apart, raise both heels off the floor so that you are on your toes. Repeat between two and ten times. As your calf muscles strengthen you should be able to stay on your toes for longer periods of time. This exercise also helps your balance.

Figure 4

Front of thigh Using a chair or wall for support, stand with your left leg in front of your right, both knees bent, your right heel off the floor. Tuck in your bottom, and move your hip forward until you feel a gentle stretch in the front of your right thigh. Now alternate legs. Repeat between two and ten times (see Figure 5).

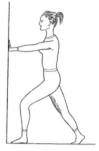

Figure 5

Back of thigh Stand with your legs slightly bent, your left leg about 20 cm (8 in) in front of your right leg. Keeping your back straight, place both hands on your hips and lean forward a little. Now straighten your left leg, tilting your bottom upwards until you feel a gentle stretch in the back of your left thigh. Now alternate legs. Repeat between two and ten times (see Figure 6).

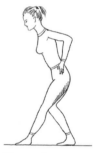

Figure 6

Groin Spreading your legs slightly, your hips facing forward and your back straight, bend your left leg and, keeping the right leg straight, move it slowly sideways until you feel a gentle stretch in your groin. Gently move to the right, bending your right leg as you straighten the left (see Figure 7).

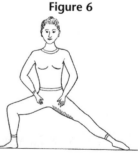

Figure 7

Chest Keeping your back straight, your knees slightly bent and your pelvis tucked under, place your arms as far behind your lower back as you can. Now move your shoulders and elbows back until you feel a gentle stretch in your chest (see Figure 8).

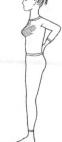

Back of upper arm With your knees slightly bent, your back straight, and your pelvis tucked under, raise your left arm and bend it so that your hand drops behind your back. Using your right hand, apply slight pressure backwards and downwards on your left arm, until you feel a gentle stretch (see Figure 9).

Figure 8

Strengthening exercises

Not all people with CFS/ME can tolerate strengthening exercises. If you think you may be able to cope with a few, don't forget to use great caution, beginning with one or two repetitions of your chosen exercises. The movements may seem easy at the time, but the real test is how you feel the next morning.

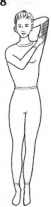

The following exercises help condition the muscles required for pushing, pulling and lifting. They will also help increase your stamina. Remember to incorporate small pauses between repetitions, to focus on staying relaxed – and don't forget to breathe as you exercise.

Figure 9

Thighs (1) The large muscles running along the top of your thigh (quadriceps) quickly grow weak with inactivity. Strengthening exercises will help you walk, climb stairs and get in and out of chairs more easily. Lean back against a wall, your feet 30 cm (12 in) away from the base of the wall, and with your posture aligned, slowly squat down, keeping your heels on the ground. (Don't go too far down at first.) Now slowly straighten your legs again. Repeat between two and ten times, lowering yourself further as, in time, your muscles strengthen.

Thighs (2) Holding on to a sturdy chair and keeping your back 'tall', bend and then slowly straighten both legs, keeping your heels on the floor. Repeat the exercise between two and ten times (see Figure 10).

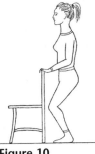

Figure 10

Thighs (3)   Sit in a chair and push your knees together. Hold for a few seconds. Repeat between two and ten times.

Upper back   Lie face down on the floor and, keeping your legs straight, gently raise your head and shoulders. Hold to a count of two, then lower. Repeat between two and ten times (see Figure 11).

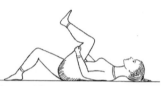

Figure 11

Lower back   Lie on your back, using a small rolled cloth to support your neck. Lift first your left leg, pulling it towards your chest until you feel a gentle pull in your bottom and lower back. Repeat with the right leg. Now pull both legs up together. Repeat each exercise between two and ten times (see Figure 12).

Figure 12

Abdomen   **(1)**   The abdominal muscles commonly grow very weak in people with CFS/ME. However, the stronger they are, the more they support your back. Lie on your back,

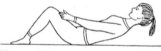

Figure 13

using a small rolled towel to support your neck. Bend your knees and place your feet flat on the floor. Now raise your head and shoulders, reaching with your arms towards your knees. Remember to keep the middle of your back on the floor (see Figure 13).

Abdomen (2)   If you are not up to doing sit-ups, the following exercise is just as effective. Lie on your back, using a small rolled cloth to support your neck. Pull in your stomach muscles and try to flatten your spine against the floor. Hold to a count of two, then release. Repeat between two and ten times.

Arms   Place your left hand on your chest and press for a few seconds. Do the same with your right arm. Repeat between two and ten times.

Push-ups   Stand with your hands flat against a wall, your body straight. Carefully lower your body towards the wall, then slowly push away. Repeat two to ten times. At first stand quite near the wall, then try moving further away as you grow stronger (see Figures 14a and 14b).

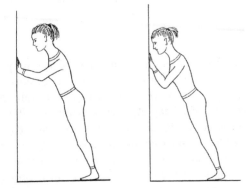

Figures 14(a) and (b)

Using small weights   People with milder symptoms may now be able to increase their strength by using small weights. The type that fasten with Velcro around the wrists and ankles are recommended. Weights of 250 g (about 8 oz) each slip into small pockets sewn into the band. (This product may be purchased at most fitness and exercise outlets.) Start by using one weight only:

1 With the armbands around your wrists, stand with your feet slightly apart. Making sure that only your upper body moves, turn carefully to the left, swinging both arms as you move. Repeat two or three times. Now perform the same exercise and number of repetitions, swinging your body and arms to the right. Ensure the movements are slow and fluid.

2 Keeping your left elbow close to your waist, slowly raise your left forearm so it almost touches your shoulder. Lower the arm until it is at right angles with your upper arm, then slowly raise again. Ensure your movements are slow and continuous.

3 Bending your left arm so that your elbow is down and your forearm upright – your wrist at your shoulder – raise your arm upward until your elbow is straight. Bring it straight back down to the original position. Repeat once more, then do the same with your right arm.

As you gain in strength and flexibility you may, first of all, be able to increase the repetitions and, second, add to the weight lifted. If your pain levels are higher than normal the next day, however, I recommend that you postpone these exercises until you feel stronger.

Low-impact aerobic activity

The following aerobic activities are listed in order of difficulty. Always ensure that you choose an aerobic exercise that you enjoy and that is within your physical and practical scope.

Walking

Walking is low-impact weight-bearing aerobic activity which aids mobility, strength and stamina and helps protect against osteoporosis. If your symptoms are severe, you may just want to walk to the nearest lamp-post and back every day until your symptoms start to stabilize. You could then walk to the second lamp-post each day for a week, then to the third lamp-post each day for a week, and so on. Walking is the easiest and most convenient aerobic activity for most people. After increasing the distance over several weeks, you may surprise yourself at how far you actually can walk.

Of course, poor weather conditions may prevent you from walking outdoors, perhaps for several weeks at a time, which makes an electric treadmill an excellent investment. This will not only give you the freedom to walk at any time you like, it can also make it possible to achieve greater distances than could be hoped for in the more uneven terrain most of us encounter outdoors. The monotony of walking on a treadmill can be overcome by positioning it near to a shelf so you can read a book or magazine at the same time. Wearing a portable audio player such as an MP3 or CD player helps to pass the time more quickly, too.

Treadmills should never wholly replace outdoor walking, however. Indeed, fresh air and sunlight are important for the following reasons:

- They help to dispel toxic gases from our bodies, via the lungs.
- Clean, fresh oxygen helps to sustain the metabolic reactions within every cell in our bodies.
- Sunlight provides our bodies with important vitamins, such as vitamin D which helps to keep our bones strong.

Stepping

Although greatly beneficial, stepping is often very difficult for people with CFS/ME. If you think you may be able to tackle it, you should start with a small step, i.e. a wide, hefty book (maybe a catalogue or a telephone directory) placed securely against a bottom stair. (After two to three weeks you may be able to use the bottom stair itself.) Place first your left foot, then your right foot onto the book/step. Now step backwards with first your left foot, then your right. Repeat between two and ten times, then alternate feet, placing first your right foot, then your left. You may eventually be able to perform the exercise for five or ten minutes.

Trampoline jogging

Jogging on a small trampoline can, if care is taken, provide good aerobic exercise. Become accustomed to the feel of it by simply lifting your heels – not your feet – as if you are walking. If you can manage to get into a rhythm, the trampoline will do much of the work for you. Continue for two or three minutes. Walking on the spot (on the trampoline) should be your next aim, and gentle jogging may eventually be achieved. Remember not to get carried away, though! Small, inexpensive trampolines are available from most exercise equipment outlets.

Aqua aerobics

Aqua aerobics, sometimes called 'aqua-cizes', can be a pleasing and beneficial alternative to swimming, which may be too difficult to tackle at first. The water supports your body as you exercise, removing the shock factor and conditioning your muscles with the minimum of discomfort. The pressure of the water also causes your chest to expand, encouraging deeper breathing and increased oxygen intake.

Rather than exercising alone in the baths, you may wish to join an aqua aerobics class. As well as providing encouragement, this can bring you into contact with people who have similar health problems. Most public swimming baths run aqua aerobics sessions, some of which are graded according to ability. You should inform the instructor of your limitations, and avoid the more taxing exercises.

Aqua aerobics, as with all types of exercise, is only truly beneficial when performed regularly. If you live a long way from the swimming baths, you will probably find yourself attending less and less, then feel angry and frustrated for eventually giving up. To avoid such feelings, be wary of undertaking activities that will be hard for you to do regularly.

Swimming

Swimming is a good all-round aerobic exercise which puts little stress on your body and works all the major muscle groups. Moreover, it puts less strain on the heart and cardiovascular system than many other aerobic activities – for example, playing a sport, running and cycling. Once again, you should only take up swimming if you can realistically get to the swimming baths easily. It also helps if you enjoy swimming.

Cycling

Whether you use a stationary or regular bicycle, cycling provides an efficient cardiovascular workout. Be cautious, though. Because of the continuous motion, your legs have no opportunity to rest as they would between most other types of exercise. Cycling can, therefore, increase your fatigue and other symptoms. It is best to start by pedalling slowly, gradually building momentum, and at first limit your sessions to two or three minutes. When your symptoms have stabilized, you may be able to gradually build up to 20 or 30 minutes. An exercise bike should always be set at a low tension.

Cooling-down exercises

Cooling down the muscles after exercise is just as important as warming them up beforehand. Again, you should choose the exercises with which you know you can cope. If all the following are beyond your scope, repeat your choice of warm-up exercises instead. The cool-down phase should last for up to five minutes.

Calf Keeping your back and right leg straight, place your palms against a wall, and bend your left knee (so that it extends further than your left ankle). Press the heel of your right foot into the floor until you feel a gentle stretch. (Move your right foot further back if you don't feel a stretch.) Now exercise the other calf in the same way.

Upper back Sitting on the floor with your knees bent, hold on to your ankles and slowly round your back. Pull in your tummy and lower your head until you feel a gentle stretch in the middle of your back.

Chest Sitting on the floor, place your hands on your lower back, moving your shoulders backwards until you feel a gentle stretch in your chest (see Figure 15).

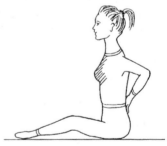

Figure 15

Back of thigh Lie on your back (using a small rolled cloth to support your neck) and bend both knees. Now raise your left leg. Placing one hand above your knee and the other below,

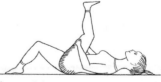

Figure 16

slowly ease the leg towards your shoulders until you feel a gentle stretch in the back of your left thigh. Now do the same with the right leg (see Figure 16).

Front of thigh Lying on your stomach, bend your left leg and hold your ankle with your nearest hand. Now, keeping your back straight, push your pelvis into the floor until you feel a gentle stretch in the front of your left thigh. Repeat the exercise with the right leg (see Figure 17).

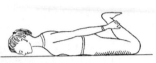

Figure 17

Abdominals Lying on your stomach, place your hands and fore-arms on the floor and slowly raise your upper body until you feel a gentle stretch in your abdominal muscles (see Figure 18).

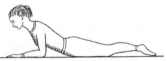

Figure 18

Getting started on your routine

It is important to set aside sufficient time to perform your exercise routine. Don't be tempted to rush because you want to see a certain TV programme.

- If you can, relax your muscles by taking a warm shower shortly after waking.
- Eat a light breakfast to boost your energy levels – you should not exercise after a heavy meal.
- Dress in loose, comfortable clothing and good, supportive training shoes.
- Ensure that exercise is carried out in a warm place.
- Start slowly and carefully. Be sure to perform only two or three rep-etitions of your chosen exercises. People with milder symptoms will be able to carry out ten repetitions sooner than people with severe symptoms.
- As you exercise, keep checking your posture. Allowing your head and shoulders to droop or your back to slacken puts added strain on your muscles. They then burn more energy, causing added pain and fatigue.
- Take care that you don't involuntarily hold your breath when exer-cising. Breathe deeply and evenly.

- Try to visualize the muscle group being exercised. This should prevent other muscle groups from being accidentally held tensely.
- Ensure that you pause between repetitions. As there is a slight delay between muscle contraction and relaxation, contracting a muscle without pause means you do so with the muscle already contracted. This causes a build-up of lactic acid in the area concerned, which in turn causes more aching and pain.
- After exercising, it is important to allow time for recovery before attempting further activity. Don't berate yourself if your fatigue and pain levels are higher than ever afterwards. Get some extra rest, then begin a toned-down version of your routine as soon as you are able.
- Don't try to make up for the days when you weren't able to do much. Set your absolute limit at the start of each session, and stick to it.
- Listen to the signals from your body. For example, if you start to feel an increase in fatigue and pain during your aerobic activity, stop immediately. Carry out your chosen cooling-down exercises, then allow your body to rest.

7

Complementary therapies

An increasing number of people with health problems are turning to complementary therapies such as acupuncture, aromatherapy and so on, often used in conjunction with their mainstream medications. If you are using or thinking of using complementary therapies, please be aware that some types can cause adverse reactions and that the quality and strength of such medication is not controlled by a regulating body. In comparison with mainstream medicine where a great deal of research has been carried out, there has been very little research and few controlled scientific trials into the effects of complementary medicine. Before deciding to use a particular therapy, try to find out as much about it as you can. You could also ask your doctor's advice.

It must be said that many people who use complementary therapies report significant benefits, perhaps some of which come from knowing they are doing something positive to help themselves. There is no doubt that the more relaxing therapies can reduce the stress caused by the symptoms of CFS/ME.

Acupuncture

An ancient form of Oriental healing, acupuncture involves puncturing the skin with fine needles at specific points in the body. These points are located along energy channels (meridians) that are believed to be blocked where allergy is present. This energy is known as chi (also spelt 'qi'). Needles are inserted to increase, decrease or unblock the flow of chi energy so that the balance of yin and yang is restored.

Yin, the female force, is calm and passive; it also represents dark, cold, swelling and moisture. On the other hand, yang, the male force, is stimulating and aggressive, representing heat, light, contraction and dryness. It is thought that an imbalance in these forces is the cause of illness and disease. For example, a person who feels the cold and suffers fluid retention and fatigue would be considered to have an excess of yin. A person suffering from repeated headaches, however, will be deemed to have an excess of yang. Emotional, physical and environmental factors are believed to disturb the chi energy balance and can also be treated. According to acupuncturists, following a healthy balanced diet, as recommended in Chapter 5, can go a long way towards restoring the balance of yin and yang, too.

In your acupuncture session, the therapist determines your particular acupuncture points – it is thought there are as many as 2,000 acupuncture points on the body and a set method is used to establish exactly where they are. At a consultation, questions may be asked about your lifestyle, sleeping patterns, fears, phobias and reactions to stress. Your pulses will be felt, after which the acupuncture itself is carried out, very fine needles being placed at the relevant sites. The first consultation will normally last for an hour, and you should notice a change for the better after four to six sessions – if not, there is really no point in carrying on.

Aromatherapy

Certain health disorders are treated by stimulating our sense of smell with aromatic oils known as *essential oils*. It is believed that such stimulation with a particular smell can help to treat a particular health problem. Indeed, there's no doubt at all that aromatherapy can aid relaxation and help to reduce the anxiety associated with CFS/ME.

Concentrated essential oils are extracted from plants and may be inhaled, rubbed directly into the skin or used in bathing. Each odour relates to its plant of origin – so lavender oil has the aroma of the lavender plant, and geranium has the aroma of the geranium plant.

Plant essences have been used for healing throughout the ages, smaller amounts being used for aromatherapy purposes than in herbal medicines. Aromatherapy oils are obtained either by steaming a particular plant extract until the oil glands burst, or by soaking the plant extract in hot oil so that the cells collapse and release their essence.

Techniques used in aromatherapy

There are several ways of using aromatherapy. The main ones are as follows:

- *Inhalation* – Giving the fastest result, the inhalation of essential oils has a direct influence on the olfactory (nasal) organs, which is immediately received by the brain. Steam inhalation is the most popular technique, carried out either by mixing a few drops of oil with a bowlful of boiling water and leaning over it to breathe in the steam, or by using an oil burner where the flame from a tea-light candle heats a small saucer of water containing a few drops of oil.

- *Massage* – Essential oils produced specifically for massage are normally pre-diluted. They should never be applied to the skin in an undiluted (pure) form. When using undiluted essential oils, mix three or four drops with a neutral carrier oil, such as olive oil, tea tree oil or safflower oil. After penetrating the skin, the oils are absorbed by the body, and this is believed to exert a positive influence on a particular organ or set of tissues. Massage is helpful in easing sore muscles, increasing circulation and relaxing tension.
- *Bathing* – Tension and anxiety can be reduced by using aromatherapy oils in the bath. A few drops of pure essential oil should be added directly to running tap water – it mixes more efficiently this way. No more than 20 drops of oil in total should be used.

Oils for relaxation

Lavender is the most popular oil for relaxation purposes. It is known to be a wonderful restorative and excellent for relieving tension headaches as well as stress. However, there are several others that either used alone or blended can provide a relaxing atmosphere – Roman chamomile and ylang ylang, for example. Ylang ylang has relaxing properties and a calming effect on the heart-rate, and can relieve palpitations and raised blood pressure. Chamomile can be very soothing, too, and aids both sleep and digestion.

Drop your relaxation oils into the vessel part of an oil burner and top up with water. Light a tea-light candle (placed beneath the burner) and try to relax while the essential oils scent the whole room and you inhale their fragrance. Such oils are safe around babies and children, as rather than being overpowering the aroma is soft and soothing.

Recipe 1

- 5 drops of lavender;
- 2 drops of Roman chamomile;
- 1 drop of ylang ylang.

Blend well and diffuse in a burner.

Recipe 2

- 8 drops of mandarin;
- 3 drops of neroli;
- 3 drops of ylang ylang.

Blend well and diffuse in a burner.

Recipe 3

- 10 drops of bergamot;
- 2 drops of rose otto;
- 3 drops of Roman chamomile.

Blend well and diffuse in a burner.

Relaxation Recipes 2 and 3 can be added to 50 cc (just under 2 fl oz) of distilled water, shaken well and used in a spray bottle for a non-toxic room-freshener with relaxing properties.

Recipe 4

For relaxation, this is a great blend for use in the bath:

- 3 drops of lavender;
- 2 drops of marjoram;
- 2 drops of basil;
- 1 drop of vetiver;
- 1 drop fennel.

Stimulating oils

The aromatherapy oils capable of stimulating mind and body, boosting the immune system and reducing fatigue include orange, rose, lavender and neroli. These oils can be mixed together in different combinations and added to a carrier oil such as tea tree oil to make massage oils.

Hypnotherapy

Hypnotherapy is commonly described as an altered state of consciousness, lying somewhere between being awake and being asleep. People under hypnosis are aware of their surroundings, yet their minds are, to a large extent, under the control of the hypnotist. The main purposes of hypnotherapy are to promote relaxation, reduce tension, increase energy and boost motivation. It also aims to increase confidence and make a person more able to cope with problems.

At a hypnotherapy session, the therapist will take a full psychological and physiological history then slowly talk you into a trance state. The therapist can either use direct suggestion – i.e. intimating that symptoms will notably lessen – or will begin to explore the root cause of any tension, anxiety or depression. The exact nature of the therapy depends largely on the problem for which treatment is being sought.

One common fear is that while the patient is in a trance the therapist may implant dangerous suggestions or extract improper personal information. I can only say that patients can come out of a trance at any time – particularly if they are asked to do or say anything they would not even contemplate when awake. And malpractice would only have to be brought to light once to ruin the therapist's career. You may prefer to visit a hypnotherapist recommended by your doctor.

There are many anecdotal reports of improvements from using hypnotherapy, but many experts say there is insufficient scientific evidence for them to promote this type of treatment. It is definitely an area worthy of further research, and it is to be hoped this takes place in years to come.

Homeopathy

The homeopathic approach to medicine is holistic – the overall health of a person, physical, emotional and psychological, is assessed before treatment commences. The practitioner will ask you about your medical history and personality traits, then offer a remedy compatible with your symptoms as well as with your temperament and characteristics. Consequently, two individuals with the same disorder may be offered entirely different remedies.

The homeopathic concept is that 'like cures like'. It is said that the full healing abilities of homeopathy were first recognized in the early nineteenth century when German doctor Samuel Hahnemann noticed that the herbal cure for malaria – which was based on an extract of cinchona bark (quinine) – actually produced symptoms of malaria. Further tests convinced him that the production of mild symptoms caused the body to fight the disease. He went on to successfully treat malaria patients with dilute doses of cinchona bark.

Each homeopathic remedy is first 'proved' by being taken by a healthy person – usually a volunteer homeopath – and the symptoms noted. This remedy is said to be capable of curing the same symptoms in an ill person. The whole idea of 'proving' and using homeopathic remedies can be difficult to comprehend, as it is exactly the opposite of how conventional medicines operate.

Although the remedies are safe and non-addictive, occasionally the patient's symptoms may worsen briefly. This is known as a 'healing crisis' and is usually short-lived. It is actually a good indication that the remedy is working well.

Case studies suggest that homeopathy can bring significant relief for most health problems; however, to date no convincing clinical research studies exist. A range of remedies can be found in most high-street chemists and online homeopathic chemists.

The remedies often used in treating CFS/ME are as follows:

- *Kali phos* for fatigue with trembling, due to stress or nervous exhaustion from overwork. Symptoms include irritability, anxiety, fear of losing control and muscle fatigue upon exertion. Take the 30c strength twice daily for up to 14 days. If beneficial, repeat the dose.
- *Arsenicum album* for exhaustion accompanied by anxiety, constant feelings of cold and joint and muscle pain, aching and burning all over from stiffness, weakness with exertion, tendency to migraines, loose bowels and blurred vision. Take the 30c strength twice daily for up to 14 days. If beneficial, repeat the dose.
- *Nux vomica* for irritable fatigue caused by lack of sleep, stress or overwork. Tense muscles, feeling chilled, joint pain and indigestion are symptoms. Take the 30c strength twice daily for up to 14 days. Repeat the dose if beneficial.
- *Argentum nitricum* for symptoms that include being fearful, anxiety-ridden and secretive, with irrational motives for your actions, which are often kept hidden. Other symptoms are: headaches with coldness and trembling, poor sleep and bad dreams. Take one dose of *Argentum nitricum* 30x or 12c three times daily, as needed for up to three days.
- *Phosphoricum acidum* for emotional and physical exhaustion and feelings of apathy. Take one dose of *Phosphoricum acidum* 30x or 15c three times daily, as needed for up to three days.
- *Picricum acidum* for feelings of exhaustion after the least exertion, especially after mental exertion, and an aversion to food. You may feel so tired that you lack willpower and determination. Take one dose of *Picricum acidum* 3c or 6x three times daily, as needed for up to three days.
- *Silicea* for headaches and exhaustion from overwork. You tend to be chilly and sensitive to cold air and often have cramps in the calves and soles of your feet. Take one dose of *Silicea* 30x or 15c three times daily, as needed for up to three days.
- *Zincum metallicum* for forgetfulness and a tendency to repeat things. You are mentally exhausted and very sensitive to noise, grind your teeth while sleeping, and may suffer from chronic constipation. Take one dose of *Zincum metallicum* 30x or 15c three times daily, as needed for up to three days.

Biofeedback

Biofeedback is a treatment technique in which people can improve physical and emotional problems by using signals from their own bodies. Physiotherapists use biofeedback to help stroke victims regain movement in paralysed muscles, and psychologists use it to help anxious clients learn to relax. Specialists in many different fields use biofeedback to help their patients cope with pain.

In the late 1960s, when the term 'biofeedback' was first coined, research showed that certain involuntary actions like heart-rate, blood pressure and brain function can be altered by tuning into the body. For instance, many people calm anxiety by reading an interesting book. As a result, their heart stops racing and their blood pressure drops to more normal levels. Later research has shown that biofeedback can help in the treatment of many conditions and that we have more control over so-called involuntary function than we once thought possible. Scientists are currently trying to determine just how much voluntary control we can exert.

Biofeedback is now widely used to treat pain, high and low blood pressure, paralysis, epilepsy and many other disorders. The technique is taught by psychiatrists, psychologists, doctors and physiotherapists.

If you have a health problem that is exacerbated by stress, a biofeedback specialist will normally teach you:

- how to use a relaxation technique;
- how to identify the circumstances that trigger (or worsen) your symptoms;
- how to cope with events you have previously avoided because of your symptoms;
- how to set attainable goals;
- how to regain control of your life.

In using biofeedback, it is important that you learn to examine your day-to-day life in order to ascertain whether you are somehow contributing to your health problem. You must recognize that you can, by your own efforts, get far more out of your life. In the correct use of biofeedback, bad habits must be changed and, most importantly, you must accept much of the responsibility for maintaining your own health.

Scientists believe that relaxation is the key to the success of this technique. You will be taught to react with a calmer frame of mind to certain stimuli – being asked to look after a young child when you feel terrible already, for example. As a result, the stress response is not triggered and adrenalin is not pumped into the bloodstream. Without biofeedback training, adrenalin may be released repeatedly, causing chronic anxiety, stress, muscle tension and depression. However, with biofeedback training it is easier to say 'no' or to take any other action necessary to protect yourself and improve your condition.

If you think you might benefit from biofeedback training, you should discuss the matter with your doctor.

Reflexology

Reflexology, an ancient Oriental therapy, was only recently adopted in the Western world. It operates on the proposition that the body is divided into different energy zones, all of which can be exploited in the prevention and treatment of any disorder.

Reflexologists have identified ten energy channels beginning in the toes and extending to the fingers and the top of the head. Each channel relates to a particular bodily zone, and to the organs in that zone. For example, the big toe relates to the head – the brain, ears, sinus area, neck, pituitary glands and eyes. By applying pressure to the appropriate terminal in the form of a small, specialized massage, a practitioner can determine which energy pathways are blocked.

Experts in this type of manipulative therapy claim that all the organs of the body are reflected in the feet. They also believe that reflexology aids the removal of waste products and blockages within the energy channels, improving circulation and lymph gland function. Reflexology is certainly relaxing – for the mind as well as the body. Indeed, as well as reducing stress, it can improve depression.

Many therapists prefer to take down a full case-history before commencing treatment. Each session takes up to 45 minutes (the preliminary session may take longer), and you will be treated sitting in a chair or lying down.

Herbal remedies

Herbal medicine is the oldest system of medicine available and remains the most widely used. Indeed, according to the World Health Organization, 80 per cent of the world's population use herbalism as their main form of treatment.

Your chosen trained herbalist will normally check your pulse rate and the colour of your tongue for clues as to which bodily organs are energy-depleted. He or she will then write a prescription for very precise doses according to your needs. Tablets made from compressed herbal extracts are often given, but you may simply receive a bag of weighed and ground dried roots, flowers and bark with which you should make an 'infusion' according to the herbalist's instructions. Herbal nerve tonics and stress-reducing adaptogens are particularly supportive of the nervous system in people with CFS/ME.

If you wish to self-prescribe two or three herbal remedies, choose from the list below, according to your symptoms. Always use herbal remedies with caution, and inform your doctor before starting treatment as they can interact with your usual chemical medications.

- *Ginkgo biloba* – This herbal antioxidant is useful for improving blood circulation. As a result, cognitive function (concentration, memory, etc.) is improved, as is energy production. As people taking prescription medication such as warfarin and aspirin can react adversely to this supplement, please consult your doctor before use. Follow the dosage instructions on the label.
- *Echinacea* – This herb has broad antibiotic properties, much like penicillin. It acts as an immune-system stimulant and is capable of strengthening cell defences. As an antiviral agent, echinacea may be used by people with CFS/ME at first indications of a cold or flu to lessen the severity. Alcohol-free tinctures are now available from most health food shops.
- *Rhodiola rosea* – This powerful nutrient belongs to the family of adaptogenic herbs, which encourage the body to adapt to stress. Research has shown that *rhodiola rosea* has a protective effect on the immune system, helps to raise energy levels and aids detoxification. It also has revitalizing properties and helps to stabilize mood swings. Take up to 180 mg daily.
- *Ashwagandha* – Also an adaptogenic herb, ashwagandha (sometimes called Indian ginseng) is an important tonic, containing a broad range of healing powers that are rare in the plant kingdom. Not only is it good for restoring energy in people with chronic fatigue, it has also been shown in research to help rejuvenate the nervous system, enhance memory and concentration and ease insomnia and stress. Take up to 750 mg daily.
- *Siberian ginseng* – This adaptogenic herb helps to increase physical endurance under stress, protects against infections and improves hormone activity. Take 4–8 g of dried root, or 20–40 ml for tincture, or 4–8 ml of fluid extract or 200–400 mg of solid extract daily.
- *St John's Wort* – This herb is probably the most successful natural antidepressant in the world. It works by increasing the action of the chemical serotonin, improving sleep and benefiting the immune

system. If you think you are suffering from depression, this may be an effective treatment. However, antidepressants prescribed by your doctor are often more beneficial.

- *Liquorice* – This tonic for the adrenal glands provides energy and helps to heal the immune system.
- *Milk thistle* – This herb provides protection for the liver against toxic damage.
- *Wild yam* – This herb is important to central nervous system function, helping to regulate the hormone imbalance occurring in CFS/ME.
- *Cleaver* – This blood-purifying herb helps to reduce swollen glands.
- *Dandelion* – This herb is an impressive liver tonic. In CFS/ME, the liver is particularly sensitive as a result of the amount of toxins it has to expel.
- *Ginger* – When used fresh, this herb boosts the digestive and circulatory systems. It relieves nausea and a sore throat, and reduces inflammation.
- *Hawthorn* – This herb is used to improve stress and insomnia.
- *Asian angelica* – This herb is a good immune-system enhancer. It also helps to reduce the symptoms of premenstrual syndrome (PMS) and the menopause.
- *Feverfew* – This herb is often used as an alternative to aspirin for the relief of muscle pains and migraine. It can also calm feverishness.
- *Basil* – Fresh basil can aid fatigue, nausea, poor digestion, headaches and anxiety.
- *Garlic* – This antioxidant herb is a great immune system booster, helping to fight inflammation and viruses.

Further reading

Burgess, M. and Chalder, T. *Overcoming Chronic Fatigue*. Constable and Robinson Publishing, London, 2005.

Campling, E. and Sharpe, M. *Chronic Fatigue Syndrome: The Facts*. Oxford University Press, Oxford, 2008.

Chalder, Trudi. *Coping with Chronic Fatigue*. Sheldon Press, London, 2002.

Craggs-Hinton, Christine. *The Chronic Fatigue Healing Diet*. Sheldon Press, London, 2003.

Gibson, I. *Inquiry into the Status of CFS/ME and Research into Causes and Treatment*. The Group on Scientific Research into Myalgic Encephalomyelitis (ME), 2006 (a report produced by a cross-party group of UK MPs: see <http://www.erythos.comgibsonenquiry/docs/ME_Inquiry_Report.pdf>).

Hale, M. and Miller, C. *The Chronic Fatigue Syndrome Cookbook; Delicious and Wellness-Enhancing Recipes Created Especially for CFS Sufferers*. Citadel Press, New York, 1997.

Marshall, Fiona. *Overcoming Tiredness and Exhaustion*. Sheldon Press, London, 2006.

Useful addresses

Action for M.E.
PO Box 2778
Bristol BS1 9DJ
Tel.: 0845 1232380 (membership); 0845 123 2314 (helpline)
Website: www.afme.org.uk

Association of Young People with ME (AYME)
10 Vermont Place
Tongwell
Milton Keynes MK15 8JA
Tel.: 08451 23 23 89 (10 a.m. to 2 p.m., Monday to Friday)
Website: www.ayme.org.uk
An online and telephone information and support organization especially for young people with the condition and their carers.

Chronic Fatigue Association of America
PO Box 220398
Charlotte
NC 28222-0398
Tel.: (+001) 704 365 2343
Website: www.cfids.org

Chronic Fatigue Research and Treatment Unit
King's College Hospital
First Floor, Mapother House
De Crespigny Park
Denmark Hill
London SE5 8AZ
Tel.: 020 3228 5075
Website: kcl.ac.uk/projects/cfs

ME Association
7 Apollo Office Court
Radclive Road
Gawcott
Bucks MK18 4DF
Tel.: 01280 818968 (9.30 a.m. to 4.30 p.m.)
Website: www.meassociation.org.uk

ME Research UK
The Gateway
North Methven Street
Perth PH1 5PP
Scotland
Tel.: 01738 451234
Website: www.meresearch.org.uk

M.E. Support
Website: www.mesupport.co.uk
An online support website founded by a person with the condition and offering information and help on all aspects of coping with ME.

National M.E. Centre
Disablement Services Centre
Old Harold Wood Hospital Site
Gubbins Lane
Harold Wood
Romford
Essex RM3 0AR
Tel.: 01708 378050
Website: www.nmec.org.uk
A telephone-based organization run by volunteer specialist support workers who offer advice and information. Ring Monday or Thursday between 11 a.m. and 1 p.m. Appointments with a specialist worker may also be arranged.

Index

activity 1, 4, 6, 22–7
    activity list 4–14
    easier ways to do things 24–7
alcohol 74
anxiety 41–3
audio equipment 31–2
awareness meditation 28

chemical sensitivities 79–80
children 4, 9, 48, 56, 59–60
Cognitive Behavioral Therapy (CBT)
    21, 45, 50
complementary therapies 95–104
    acupuncture 95–6
    aromatherapy 96–8
    biofeedback 101–2
    herbal remedies 102–4
    homeopathy 99–100
    hypnotherapy 98–9
    reflexology 102

deep breathing 29–30
diet and nutrition 62–81
    wholefood diet 63–7
    cow's milk products 67–8
    foods to avoid 71–3
    food elimination 75–6

emotions 12–13, 43–61
endorphins 9, 82
energy 1–14
exercise 7, 82–94
    aerobic activity 90–94
    mobility exercises 84–5
    strengthening exercises 87
    stretching exercises 85–7
    warm up exercises 83
    weights 89

fatigue 2, 9, 19, 62
fibromyalgia 31

insomnia 38–42
irrational feelings 49–51

joint mobility 1, 5, 82

limits 4

muscle tone 5
music 11–12, 32

naps 36–8
negative thinking 48–51
nutritional supplements 76–95
    5–HTP 41

occupational therapy 8
other people 45–8, 52–5

pacing 1–6, 15–27
pacing chart 7–14
patience 18
planning 24
'push and crash' cycle 18–19

reactions 15–18
rest 28–42

self-care 6–7, 10, 16
self-talk 20
sitting 25–6
sleep 28–42
smoking 74
Social Services 8, 60
special occasions 20, 22, 50
stamina 5, 13, 57–8, 69, 87

vitamin D3 41

water 80–81